PAINTING AND THE INNER WORLD

T0187655

ADRIAN STOKES

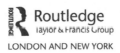

Routledge
Taylor & Francis Group

LONDON AND NEW YORK

First published in 1963 by
Tavistock Publications (1959) Limited

Reprinted in 2001 by
Routledge
2 Park Square, Milton Park, Abingdon, Oxon, OX14 4RN

Simultaneously published in the USA and Canada by Routledge

711 Third Avenue, New York, NY 10017

Transferred to Digital Printing 2007

Routledge is an imprint of the Taylor & Francis Group

First issued in paperback 2013

British Library Cataloguing in Publication Data
A CIP catalogue record for this book
is available from the British Library

Painting and the Inner World
ISBN 978-0-415-26491-4 (hbk)
ISBN 978-0-415-84981-4 (pbk)

ADRIAN STOKES

Painting
and the
Inner World

Including a dialogue with
DONALD MELTZER, M.D.

TAVISTOCK PUBLICATIONS

First published in 1963
by Tavistock Publications (1959) Limited
2 Park Square, Milton Park,
Abingdon, Oxon, OX14 4RN
in 11pt. Times Roman
by C. Tinling and Co. Ltd.,
Liverpool, London and Prescot

To Telfer

Contents

Contents

Acknowledgements

In regard to Turner, I would record the help and kindness of the Keeper, Department of Prints and Drawings, British Museum, and of his staff; my very particular gratitude to Mr. Martin Butlin, Assistant Keeper at the Tate Gallery. Mr. Charles M. W. Turner kindly allowed me to study his collection. I am further indebted to Mr. Lawrence Gowing and to Mr. David Sylvester for their interest and most useful advice.

A.S.

I. PAINTING AND THE INNER WORLD

I. Painting and the Inner World

There is room in the outside world for everybody's mental furniture to be rearranged. The artist is most convinced of it, but we are all psychical removal men on shorter hours: we are surprised to see arm-chairs and desks in the street before a second-hand shop; it is as if a *tromp-l'oeil* art had revealed an entire unconscious, without any aid from symbolism, without requiring imagery from a transposition.

Since we are removal men who sit down to look over their work, there is no problem concerning the contemplative character of the so-called aesthetic emotion, much canvassed in aesthetics since Kant. The inner world, indeed, perpetually forces its imprint of a symbol upon *all* perception; but art devotes itself entirely to sense-data, to every significance attaching to them, in order to focus steadily on integration of the inner world as an outer image.

Art, therefore, is a refinement upon an unceasing affective occurrence. Those averse to art expatiate upon the inner world through other activities, possibly in a manner far less testing. Art aims a blow at some forms of respectability and often provides a converse to comfort distributed by keepsakes and knick-knacks, by the preference for at least one kind of vulgarity (that sometimes serves to exclude others). A Sung bowl renders no doggy acquiescence: we must come to terms: it does not live up to us and it has lost in our eyes, or largely lost, the emblematic-cultural qualities from which it will have been fashioned. Yet the necessity remains to found art in common experience and the artist in common man. Viewed historically, the separation of the artist from the artificer, of the artificer from the ordinary man, and even

3

of technological advances from aesthetic value, appear to be recent developments. The emergence of the artist as we now think of him implies what will seem to some a wayward emphasis upon the inner life, since our epoch cannot dare to view its technological excesses as symbols of the psyche in a deep sense, nor, consequently, much else that is made.

There is nothing surprising, therefore, that a display which was taken by them to be evidence of the tractable tameness of art, accorded with the wishes of many people who formerly used to crowd into the Academy summer exhibition; they found there illusionist models of careless perception free of deep-set principles of structure, and so of acute reference to the inner life. But those who avoid contemplation even of Nature, are likely to have over-strong defensive attitudes against contact with their inner world, attitudes of denial fortified by holidays in droves, by the reading of the Sunday paper in a closed car parked at a beauty spot, by transistor sets that drown the beach's surf. In such experiences that allow not even for her conquest in an active sense, Nature whose contemplation, whose close presence, mirrors the forms of an inner self, becomes enslaved to transistor-inspired identifications that reduce character to complacent terms. It is one lure of the circus wherein a conscious theme, other than the conventionalized *Haute École*, is the victory over four-legged beasts who, however clumsily and pain-fully, have been trained to ape their masters. Man celebrates still the conquest of beasts: it would be astonishing, were not beasts equated with what in himself he cannot supervise with comparable satisfaction, and would deny.

Artist or aesthete, on the other hand, cultivates some admitted inflections at least in the outer of the inner world. The artist is under compulsion to repair the inner world in terms of co-ordinating projections upon the outer. A coher-ence discovered in the meaning of sense-data, innocent of any justification such as the usefulness of the perception, corresponds, he feels, to the gratuitous force, as it will sometimes appear, of his reparative aim. Everyone deplores ugliness and chaos not only for the actual losses they portend but because they are referred to inner losses, inner disarrangement. The reaction on the part of the artist to this inner reference does not always evoke from him a drive for neatness, tidiness, cleanliness: he may hold such more narrowly obsessional glosses in some contempt, may even regard them too as a form of poverty, as thin denial of an evil that lies beneath, dead or dying things that lack help from wider reparative effort.

It seems desirable that I give a precise account of what I mean by the inner world, the one of Freud and Melanie Klein. Apart from the fact that I claim no precise picture, there is always the difficulty that the concepts of psychoanalysis are little known and far less understood, yet it is impossible to interpolate several treatises available elsewhere.

The aspect of the psyche that most concerns our context is the potential chaos and the attempts to achieve stability whether predominantly through defences of splitting such as getting rid of parts of the psyche on to other people, or through denial, omnipotence, idealization, or whether predominantly by the less excluding method, the prerogative of the truly adult being, that entails recognition of great diversity in the psyche under the aegis of trust in a good object. The word 'object' may seem obscure but it is used with determination. By means of introjection, the opposite of projection, the ego has incorporated phantasy figures (and part-figures such as the breast) both good and bad. These are objects to us not only because they have come from without but because they can retain within the psyche their phantasied corporeal character. The ego itself may be much split: many parts may have been projected permanently to inhabit other people in order to control them, an instance—it is called projective identification—of the interweaving of outer and

5

inner relationships. Though this phantasy-commerce be deeply buried in our minds, it colours, nevertheless, as I have indicated, the reception of sense-data in much-transposed terms. Form in art, I have urged elsewhere, reconstitutes the independent, self-sufficient, outside good object, the whole mother whom the infant should accept to be independent from himself, as well as the enveloping good breast of the earliest phase, at the foundation of the ego, the relationship with which is of the merging kind. In this reparative act the attempt must be made to bring less pleasing aspects of these objects to bear, parallel with the integrative process in the ego as a whole that art mirrors no less. (Stokes, 1947, 1951, 1955a, 1955b, 1958, 1961).

Furthermore, within a pattern of integration, there intrude narrow compulsive traits both of offence and defence in sublimated forms. We are likely to observe an obsessional aspect of art within the broad compulsion to repair and to integrate what has been threatened, scattered, or destroyed. Indeed, it is a narrower compulsive element—we shall find it in Turner—that bestows on much art a quality of urgency and inevitability, causing the spectator to feel that a rigid driving force, having attained aesthetic sublimation, becomes most impressive partly because art is never to be divorced, within its limits, from truth and understanding, and partly because a successful sublimation of obsessional attitudes subject to the major conspectus, signifies that some degree of aesthetic (i.e. integrative) employment has been won from tendencies often hostile to any integrative role.

There would be nothing to art could it be exercised in despite of temperament. Not even the framework ordained by culture can be used to contrive for aesthetic expression a rule of thumb: though his working in a settled style will cloak it thickly, the artist has needed his temperament. He may work all his life within a strict convention: on the other hand, a few of the greatest European painters have manifestly

6

rediscovered, re-allocated, more and more of themselves in the terms of their art: their discoveries and extensions of themselves have ensued directly from further aesthetic exploration. Art is built directly upon previous art, indirectly upon the artist's courage about himself and about his surroundings. The student today builds little by rote that he can subsequently dismember, enlarge, and rebuild: he attempts an unprecedented immediacy of expression: the close of an evolution is tried at the beginning. I believe the fruitfulness to be limited as a rule. This is the context for the appreciation of Turner in Part III.

To return to inner objects. There will have been many visitors to Rome and to the Vatican who will have found daring shapes insistent beside the traffic roar, mingling with the contrasted movements in a street. The painted forms from galleries survive, enter and inhabit the city. The palpable images that we saw welling out of walls and canvasses, touch us profoundly because they reflect figures in ourselves, incorporated figures, whose inner presence is more variable and far less orderly. We relish it that inner tensions be transformed into the outer corporeality of contrasted attitudes amid the simulated breadth of the outside world. For a few people, at any rate, there is a related perception of dreams from which only a limited anxiety remains, a similarity with the salient impressions of shape planted in our minds by Roman sight-seeing; in regard to dreams, that is, whose content we cannot at once recall. Some people may have an impression from the dream, none the less, of density perhaps, or of great space, or of a dominant form: in effect, of an epitome in the terms of substance and space. I call it an epitome because I have found that when this impression has become the surviving imprint, yet, when later, the dream has been recalled in some detail, the sensation of an arrangement of forms had been broken up into this recall, as if these formal elements had synthesized or resolved the contradictions of the content into something not only simple but tangible. Owing to the corporeal nature of the adult's inner objects, it seems that a dream can deposit a residue of sensations of shape, as does art, the more general, and therefore less painful, though not altogether distorted, perception of inner objects.

Much visual art is founded in accumulated designations of outer character and the world of space. This conscious aim provides transcendental dimensions for the inner world, in a concrete form. We do not usually associate the word 'transcendental' with a condition expressly concrete, but it is surely admissible in the case of some methods of outer contemplation, and particularly of art that offers a single object to the senses, a version of inner objects available as one interaction. Inner idols, hated and loved, together with some of the defences or rituals they impose, are compounded. Though the subject-matter of a painting be what the theologians call carnal beauty, in so far as the picture is a work of art, the particular erotic stimulus—no painted flowers seem to have scent, no aesthetic apple cause mouths to water—becomes secondary to a more general awareness of availability that has been heightened rather than dominated by the manifest erotic content. But it is understandable to mistake or to resist the point of art, to find in its scentless flowers no suggestion but of their deadness, at any rate when naturalistic art has been considered as the only norm.

It follows from what has already been said that the inner world encountered under the aegis of aesthetic form, elicits relationships to the basic good objects, namely the self-subsistent mother and the enveloping good breast or part-object. Just as an integrated psyche reads and tempers experience by the light of a firm trust in the relationship to these good objects, so the manifold expressiveness of art, in virtue of its form, figures within their orbit; the wider the expressiveness the better, as a rule, inasmuch as aesthetic form obtains significance from the varied material to be unified of the artist's temperament, of his culture and of his inheritance from art, as well as from his subject-matter. We spectators, prepared to view the modern work of art as a good object, may contemplate in this manner an aspect of our own culture that is anything but good, yet we would not need recourse to denial or to other defence. As is well known, the artist is both the leader and the servant of his time. He is able in some degree—only some degree—in accordance with a new cultural theme or accentuation, to lend himself to the expression of a psychical position that under other aesthetic circumstances (in accordance with other cultural circumstances) might or might not have been available to him. We can have no conviction whatsoever concerning the way that even the greatest of artists would have worked had they lived in other periods. The artist's perspicacity about culture, about what upholds, destroys or ameliorates his society and his art, provides both a condition and an earnest of his truthful comment upon the inner world that he finds reflected while examining any outer situation. It is in line with the common disposal of feeling by means of projection, employed aesthetically for the purpose of insight in regard to both the within and the without and their relationship: otherwise the artist would achieve no integration, no art.

This brings me to the subject of bad objects, of aggression, of envy, of all that is negative. Again, these drives, and the objects imbued with them, could not figure in art—and they figure prominently—except under the sign of co-ordination, of the form in art that stems from the presence of good objects. Tragic art, to be so, must bear nobility. But many appreciators today seem to find it more exciting if formal elements can be observed barely to survive a monstrous expression of, say, greed. What is entirely negative or chaotic, or merely unfeeling, can never be art, and what is near to it is never great art.

9

I myself often regret that the model, as such, may appear to be obliterated by a painter's omnipotent handling in work of a predominantly representational style; by his attack, particularly in the case of a nude, since we will probably entertain the notion of a sadistic intercourse without the sense that it has been integrated; of a conflagration or annihilation, even though, in virtue of pattern, shape and colour, we are aware that something has not only been saved from the wreckage, but unified, so that the wreckage itself has become a perilous richness. Modern central European artists especially have been noted for this bravura, characteristic of what is called Expressionist art.

If it appears also as a more decorative kind of representational art, there exists a world of difference between the superb liberties that Matisse took in his painting of models and the cloudy stick of opalescent colour that Matthew Smith inflicted, especially upon his nudes. Here may sometimes—but not always—be found, grandiloquently told, a wealth made useless, a luxury without repletion, movement without a centre. The artist has seized upon a pose and almost painted the object out, that is to say, the symbol of a presence. It is possible that such opinions are a way of suggesting that Matthew Smith was, in a strict sense, but a moderate draughtsman, without entire reverence for the subtleties of figurative three-dimensional construction within the convention of which he worked; without the appreciation that this structure should initially involve (allied though it must be with the modeller's masterful handling), of the independent object in its own space, separate from the self as well as at the self's disposal. Smith's flourishings *alone*—not so Turner's we shall find—often overthrew separateness. He employed an exaggerated chiaroscuro pictorially to overpower a powerful model with an aggression that seems to me to lack much combination from florid love, unlike the Baroque painters who used this weapon. His handling, while it provides a rich

10

co-ordination—there is *some* florid love—in general sub-
stitutes itself as the object for the model, for her virtue as
the symbol of a presence, external and internal, a tendency
of modern painting that is questionable only in the naturalistic language. The abstractions and total distortions of *avant-
garde* painting and sculpture are often the means of avoiding
the problem altogether: hence the perfection of its best
achievements somewhat in the manner of music and
architecture.

Like the dominant impressions gained from Rome, we
possess in some abstract art an intense figuration for the con-
course of corporeal inner objects (and for the restored outer
object), though divorced in this case from the significance of
their attachment to precise and self-subsistent models from
the outside world: and it may well be that in common with
most image-making, exaggeration and distortion in modern
representational art has proceeded less from aggression
than from the need to describe inner states as far as possible
as such, in an outer form. But Matthew Smith, together with
other English painters of his time, often preferred not so
much to re-fashion, as masterfully to override, the model:
we glimpse her most sensationally like a martyr among the
flames: those are her bounty, for, of course, we have bounty
from art, though it is by no means always entirely pleasant.
Much painting communicates a richness, a voluptuousness,
by means of greedy, masterful attitudes that borrow for their
qualification as art the co-ordination of adult feeling. I do
not doubt that this is often most popular among those who
can 'take' it, even, and perhaps especially, among aesthetes,
or that it provides a common appliance by which the envelopment aspect of the aesthetic experience may be magnified. For, inasmuch as a part of negative feeling is commonly less integrated, being entrenched in retrograde and
split-off positions, a handling of paint that little expresses
love in its attack, is likely to bestow upon the object made,

11

and/or the object represented, a part-object flavour, though there must survive as well the opposite co-ordination inseparable from aesthetic value. This role assigned to aggression in art, also the enveloping aspect of form in general, has some connections with an inchoate or unlimited value that transports the 'soul' (whose fund of feeling is equally vast), attributed by some aesthetic theories between Addison and Kant to what was called 'the sublime', a value that came to be opposed, particularly in the guise of contemplated terror and discomfort by Burke in his treatise of 1756 or 1757, to 'a composure of the parts' reserved for the character of beauty, more connected, it seems, with self-sufficiency than with the overwhelming or enveloping character of a part-object.

Of course we must expect, and desire, aggression to figure prominently in art, so as to be integrated there. We shall find it in Turner, but not at all in the terms of an omnipotence, I would be glad to own a Matthew Smith. I am certain, however, that he was by no means a great painter, and consider that his example is unlikely to be inspiring. He often achieved vibrancy, *forcing* upon his art an immaturity, it seems to me, of libidinal feeling: the large-handedness appear spurious when compared with the more generous flourish—generous to the objects depicted—of Smith's Baroque ancestors whose curving line envelops us also. Some 'powerful', straining artists provide a caution concerning the nature of art: ambivalence will not be aesthetically resolved in terms of its waywardness but by an integration that holds the negative as such within view. Great artists, still in terms of aesthetic co-ordination and even of beauty, have shown that behind and beyond aggression there stretches the domain of refusal and of death.

What has usually happened to the co-ordinating factor in this circumstance of stress for the good object? Burke announced in the eighteenth century that sublimity, where it engenders delight—this includes art—involves a 'tranquillity

12

tinged with terror'. I think we must refer to a similar situation many noble styles, stylizations and systems of proportion, withdrawn, ideal and generalized, that can subsume a forthright expressiveness. If, as some people say, a circle is beautiful, or any geometrical figure, they can but mean that beauty resides in the delineation of such a figure on its ground: unlike the idea of circularity, an actual circle is inconceivable without the ground it modifies. I believe we should pay homage not so much to the beauty as to the feeling of order inspired in us by such remote and impersonal figures that dominate, as do the formal elements in art, the often gross particularity of their *mise-en-scène*. Formal authority, we have seen, is exercised in the universal context of ambivalence: it serves in art as an affirmation of generalized, of the least threatened, and therefore of the minimum, the safest, idea of structure. Certainly even the triangle can be broken up into lines, but perhaps the very impersonality protects, so that the identity of these minimum structures surmounts all but the most violent splitting. It is not unknown in the case of a psychotic child for all his objects to be reduced to numbers and to geometric forms. (Diatkine, 1960). A reliance upon a minimum yet regular object may well characterize the compulsive aspect of the mathematical or musical prodigy, more certainly of *idiots savants*.

But in spite of the analogies, and even comparisons, with the reduced objects of psychotic defences, I do not for a moment wish to suggest that what I call here the minimum object in art is predominantly the outcome of denial and splitting; on the contrary, the virtue in art of such wide regularity is the capacity to engage contents at loggerheads with each other, or those impossible to reconcile with a less abstracted kind of order based upon the trust in goodness. There comes about in this way stability and safety. True enough, a degree of bare formulation is the prime instrument in art of echo, of pattern and so of *any* co-ordination; it is

13

the means as well for linking expressiveness. Moreover, painting and sculpture will have been much influenced by the formal conditions of music, and particularly of architecture. But when I consider the durability of many aesthetic structures, I want to make a further connection with a safety imputed to the ego and to the reconstituted object *under all circumstances*. Though at the same time outside objects be delineated, we have seen that the comprehensive yet acceptable mode for recording the pressure of the inner life belongs especially to the part of the construction dependent upon what might be called faceless shapes. We do not, and must not, have in graphic art perfect geometry, but we often need indications of regularity, in terms of pattern and echo, that predispose us to search for suggestions of the simplest geometric figures to which so much subtlety and variety seems to have accrued, inasmuch as descriptiveness of the outside world has here bestowed the element of particularity. Art is warm, intimate, yet steadied by the tremendous safeguard of owning a quality that in isolation would be impersonal and withdrawn. While describing a figure, an artist searches for the larger, the simpler organization that, in the case of a nude, may overlap even such prominent shapes as the breasts. We are often then powerfully aware of a lively significance based upon a skeletal strength, whereas the abstractions employed in other disciplines can rarely be felt to underlie the reconstitution of a particular situation with a comparable thoroughness.

A good drawing may be lascivious, but the artist will have noted the cold facts, for instance the position of the navel in respect to the nose (of course, there is a sense in which this is not a cold fact), the relationship of key points in regard to vertical and horizontal lines. The character of the pose depends upon a suspicious exactness in such matters, upon a power to dismiss the model, to see her for some of the purposes of draughtsmanship as made up of flat patterns.

14

Thus, an aspect of the draughtsman's talent, meaningless by itself, is his facility to see a hand not as a hand but as areas of tone from which he extracts the pattern, the proportions, as well as the effect of relief, wider truths of its appearance that serve also in this kind of drawing to mirror an aspect of the inner world. These impersonal-seeming preoccupations, together with the austere or 'geometric' elements of design in general contribute to the resistant armature of the aesthetic object. During another part of the act of drawing—it should of course be exercised at the same time—when the artist makes marks for the folds of the stomach, say, he is likely in phantasy to be digging into it. I find it difficult to see how these attitudes could more than co-exist, in that they illumine each other through their co-ordination, did not one of them spell out the impervious endurance I have described under the name of a minimum object.

But not every artist—and no artist all the time—has taken full advantage of the hardiness latent in design and pattern: not every artist predominantly grasps or twists his object while trusting to this safeguard. My oldest contention in this field is that differences of approach between carving and modelling characterize pictorial conceptions as well as conceptions in all the other visual arts. (Stokes, 1932, 1935, 1937, 1949.) The carver, in a manner more nearly concrete, is jabbing into a figure's stomach. The compensatory emotion is his reverence for the stone he consults so long: he elicits meaning from a substance, precious for itself, whose subsequent forms made by the chisel were felt to be pre-existent and potential: similarly in painting there is the canvas, the rectangular surface and the whiteness to fructify, a pre-existent minimum structure that not only will be gradually affirmed but vastly enriched by the coalescence with other meanings. What a contrast, this side of art, to the summary, omnipotent-seeming aspect of creativeness, to the daring, the great daring and plastic imposition that are even more

15

characteristic and far more easily recognized and applauded, qualities that cause us to clutch at them, or that tend to envelop us.

But it has also always been my contention that some exercise of both approaches must figure in visual art. Nevertheless, the greatest exponents since the Renaissance of the rare type of painting that reveres outside objects for themselves, almost to the exclusion of projecting on to them more than the corresponding self-sufficient inner objects, have had the least, or else the tardiest, recognition of their supremacy. Those immense heroes of painting, Piero della Francesca, Georges de la Tour, Vermeer (Gowing, 1952), were forgotten and rediscovered only in the last hundred years at a time when texture, the heightened expressive use of the *matière* of painting, a substitute for pleasures in past ages available from buildings, was much on the increase. Their rediscovery, then, points to the connection between this care for material and a non-grasping approach in general, since it is not at all the surface or texture of paintings by these Old Masters that most characterizes, in their case, the 'carving' attitudes to objects.

I end invoking Piero, de la Tour, and Vermeer since it may be opportune to re-assert, in line with much I have written before and with the paper by Dr. Segal (1952 and 1955), that whatever the projection of narrow compulsions to which I have referred, whatever the primitive and enveloping relationships that ensue, the reconstitution or restoration of the outside and independent whole object (expressive equally of co-ordination in the ego) whether founded entirely, or less founded, upon what I have called minimum or generalized or ideal and impersonal conceptions, remains a paramount function in art.

16

References

BURKE, E. *A Philosophical Enquiry into the Origin of our Ideas of the Sublime and Beautiful* (ed. J. T. Boulton, London, 1958).

DIATKINE, R. 'Reflections on the Genesis of Psychotic Object Relationship in the Young Child' (*Int. J. Psycho-Anal.*, 1960).

GOWING, L. *Vermeer* (London, 1952).

MONEY-KYRLE, R. E. *Man's Picture of his World* (London, 1961).

READ, H. 'Beauty and the Beast'. *Eranos-Jahrbuch*, XXX (Zürich, 1962).

SEGAL, H. 'A Psycho-Analytical Approach to Aesthetics' (*Int. J. Psycho-Anal.*, 1952 and in *New Directions in Psycho-Analysis*, London, 1955).

STOKES, A. *The Quattro Cento* (London, 1932).

STOKES, A. *Stones of Rimini* (London, 1935).

STOKES, A. *Colour and Form* (London, 1937 and 1946).

STOKES, A. *Inside Out* (London, 1947).

STOKES, A. *Art and Science* (London, 1949).

STOKES, A. *Smooth and Rough* (London, 1951).

STOKES, A. *Michelangelo* (London, 1955a).

STOKES, A. 'Form in Art' in *New Directions in Psycho-Analysis* (London, 1955b).

STOKES, A. *Greek Culture and the Ego* (London, 1958).

STOKES, A. *Three Essays on the Painting of our Time* (London, 1961).

II. CONCERNING THE SOCIAL BASIS OF ART

Donald Meltzer, M.D.
in a Dialogue with Adrian Stokes

II. Concerning the Social Basis of Art

MELTZER:

You have asked me to amplify what I said in our conversations that followed your paper *Painting and the Inner World* (Similar to Part I of this book), read to the Imago Group.

As a practising psycho-analyst I shall draw from clinical and theoretical knowledge the implications of Melanie Klein's discoveries, with the aim of adding to what has already been written by Dr. Segal and yourself. On that foundation I shall try to extend understanding of the relationship between the artist and his viewer: hence, more widely, my concern, in this dialogue with you, will be the social value of art from the psycho-analytic angle. But first I shall want to comment on art as a therapy for the artist, especially in regard to one of the themes of your paper.

Freud, and other writers following his lead, considered artistic creativity to be a part of mental functioning very closely related to dream formation. They have explained the manner in which artistic creativity, like the dream, is taken up with a working over in the unconscious of the residues of daily experiences, particularly those of the repressed unconscious. The Kleinian approach to art has tended to emphasize a more systematic self-therapeutic process of working over and working through the basic infantile conflicts that go on in the depths in relation to internal objects. The most constructive part of this process attempts to build a firmer passage from the paranoid-schizoid to the depressive position by way of internal object relations, consolidating, stabilizing the internal world.

21

STOKES:

Before you go on, I think you must supply an account of what is meant by the paranoid-schizoid and the depressive positions.

MELTZER:

Since later on in this dialogue some implications will be drawn from Melanie Klein's formulation of the two positions, I shall restrict myself at this point to a brief differentiation between the concept of *position* and the other, more clearly developmental, concepts of *phase* and *primacy*, formulated by Freud.

Freud conceived his meta-psychology to have four aspects, topographic, genetic, dynamic and economic. Among the genetic phenomena he discovered developmental sequences that seemed to be biologically based (though open to environmental modification), centred on the shifting of primacy between erogenous zones, oral, anal, phallic and genital, as the libidinal organization of the infant and child developed. The discovery of the focal office of the Oedipus complex directed attention to *phases* of development, pre-oedipal, the period of oedipal conflict dominance, latency, puberty, adolescence, maturity, climacteric and senescence.

Melanie Klein's formulation of two *positions* does not conflict with these concepts. The emphasis lies with the organization of the self, together with the value systems involved in object relations. The formulation is only secondarily genetic in its reference, since progress from the paranoid-schizoid to the depressive position (or regressions in the opposite direction) fluctuate throughout the course of life: the transition is never complete.

The essence of the transition is twofold: on the one hand there is the struggle towards integration of self and objects, especially internal objects, whereby splitting and exclusively part-object relations are overcome in favour of integration of the self and of whole-object relations characterized by the

22

separate and self-contained qualities imputed to objects. The transition requires as well a shift in values from the preoccupation with *comfort, gratification and omnipotence* characteristic of the paranoid-schizoid organization, to the central theme of *concern* for the safety and freedom of the good objects, particularly again, internal ones, and especially the mother, her breasts, her babies and her relationship to the father.

While this shift in value systems has a link with Freud's distinction of primary and secondary process in mental functioning, it is by no means synonymous with it. Another item of importance, however, presents an identity of concept, though the form is expanded. Freud's categories of anxiety and guilt find expression in Kleinian theory with the conception of two spectra of mental pain, the persecutory anxieties of the paranoid-schizoid position and the depressive anxieties such as guilt, shame, remorse, longing etc.

Now you will recall that in conversation, talking about your concept of a minimum object, we found ourselves involved in a discussion that turned out to be an investigation of the difference between what might be called 'safety' in one's internal relationships as against 'security'. I put forward to you something that I think is inherent in Mrs. Klein's work. There is no such thing as safety in object relationships to be found in the quality of the object itself. In contrast to processes characteristic of the schizoid position in which idealization, for instance, attempts to remove the object from the realm of interpersonal processes, subject to envy and jealousy, or where the splitting mechanisms attempt to reduce an object to a point where the impulse to attack it and fragment it further, is diminished; in contrast to these mechanisms of the paranoid-schizoid position, the very heart of the depressive position is the realization that security can only be achieved through responsibility. Responsibility entails integration, that is, accepting responsibility for psychical

c

reality, for the impulsivity and affects and attitudes, for all the
different parts of the self *vis-à-vis* internal and external objects.
Inherent in the concept of the depressive position is the realization that the drive towards integration is experienced as love
for an object, that is, as the experience of cherishing the wel-
fare of an object above one's own comfort. It is also implicit
in these theories that, for an object to be loved, it must be
unique and it must have qualities of beauty and goodness
which are able to evoke in the self the feelings of love and
devotion. The corresponding inner object that undergoes
a development parallel with the self's integration, achieves
those qualities as it becomes fully human in complexity.
Thus it demands a life of its own, freedom, liberty of action,
and the right of growth and development. In relation to such
an object the feeling of love arises; the impulse, the desire,
is aroused to take responsibility for all those parts of the self
that are antagonistic and dangerous to the object. In essence
this is the basis of the drive towards integration, towards the
integrating of the various parts of the self. It perhaps is also
important to mention that love for the truth becomes very
strongly allied to the capacities to appreciate the beauty and
the goodness of the object, since manic defences, and through
them the danger of regression to the paranoid-schizoid
position, have their foundations in an attack on the truth.

I think that, in so far as the creative process is an entirely
private one, we have learned from Dr. Segal and yourself
that we should think of the artist to be representing in his
art work, as through his dreams, the continuous process of the
relationships to his internal objects, including all the vicis-
situdes of attack and reparation. But if we say that the artist
performs acts of reparation through his creativity we must
recognize that in the creative process itself, phases of attack
and phases of reparation exist in some sort of rhythmical
relationship. This implies that the artist, at any one moment
of time in the creative process, finds his objects to be in a

24

certain state of integration or fragmentation; he consequently experiences a relative state of integration or fragmentation within the infantile components of his ego in relation to his objects. It must be recognized that this process necessarily involves great anxiety. In referring to anxiety we must remember that we have in mind the whole range of persecutory and depressive anxieties.

STOKES:

You are going on to speak of the role of projective identification in regard to art. Before you begin, I would like to comment on what you have said about the plain projective character. My paper, the context for this discussion, is concerned with the ordinary projection of inner objects (though I had something to say as well about the strong projection into us of haunting shapes). You accepted it as our point of departure for this discussion, with one important exception, in the matter of what I called 'a minimum object', a phrase by which I drew attention to the bare, generalized, sometimes almost geometric, and in general, ideal, plane on which much artwork takes place. In the interests of the fight for integration, characteristic of the depressive position, about which, in accordance with Hanna Segal's formulation, we entirely agree that it provides the *mis-en-scène* for aesthetic creation, you object strongly to a mechanism in art, as seen by me, that forges safety for the object. You have just said, very notably: 'There is no such thing as safety in object relationships to be found in the quality of the object itself. In contrast with processes characteristic of the paranoid-schizoid position in which idealization, for instance, attempts to remove the object from the realm of inter-personal processes, subject to envy and jealousy, or in which the splitting mechanisms attempt to reduce an object to a point where the impulse to attack it and fragment it further is diminished; in contrast with these mechanisms of the paranoid-schizoid position, the very heart

25

of the depressive position is the realization that security can only be achieved through responsibility', i.e. for 'all the different parts of the self *vis-à-vis* internal and external objects.'

I am very far from wanting to quarrel with that statement, as you know. But you have gone on to say that art mirrors the *struggle* for integration and for an integrated object; and that there are alternations of integrated and unintegrated states in the very process of making art. No one can doubt for a moment that a trend towards idealization characterizes much of the greatest art (nor the aggressive projections against which idealization is one defence). I think that a large part of the reassurance provided by art exists in the service won from paranoid-schizoid mechanisms—the transition is never complete, you have said—for what is, overall, a triumph of integration on the depressive level. Even in the best integrated people, something, at least, of the earlier mechanisms remains active, in satisfactions as well as in the conflicts. Indeed the primitive identifications, with an oral basis, that tie society, are always particularly to the fore. The fact that you are going on to speak of the relevance to art of the primitive mechanism of projective identification among others, makes me chary of cutting any ground from under foot in the matter of early mechanisms and the production of art. Now, in *Envy and Gratitude* Melanie Klein wrote that it is not always possible to distinguish absolutely between the good and the idealized breast. Someone has said that art brings together the real and the perfect. This is not primarily a question of sugaring the pill of reality as Freud, I think, suggested the role of form to be in clothing the artist's day-dream, since to this element of invitation as he saw it, we attribute a far more fundamental part in the chemistry of the pill. All the same, art can easily be debased into a sugar-coated product that usually has great popularity among those who are hostile to art for whatever reason.

26

MELTZER:

I think Mrs. Klein was stressing the fact that only by knowing the genesis of an object can we be certain of its value. The clinical material that I shall present will demonstrate it. First, as you have indicated, I want to talk about the concept of projective identification. This is an essential concept of Melanie Klein's work, very different from the earlier Freudian concept of a projection concerned primarily with ideas, impulses, affects and attitudes. Mrs. Klein's concept defines the mental process by which very concretely portions of the self and internal objects are projected into objects in the outer or the inner world. She emphasized both the normal and pathological uses of projective identification, stressing what she called 'excessive' projective identification, excessive in so far as it was primarily sadistic and destructive in intent, or excessive in so far as it was so dedicated to the search for freedom from anxiety and pain as to interfere with the normal working through of conflicts. Bion, on the other hand, has described, particularly in his recent Congress paper, the role of projective identification in communication; he has brought this concept to the fore as the mechanism of primitive *preverbal* communication. However, since we are talking about art, we mustn't restrict this aspect to *non-verbal* modes of communication. Projective identification plays a part in *verbal* communication also where it transcends the syntactic mechanisms for transmitting information, information, that is, in the mathematical sense. What is communicated by this mechanism is the *state of mind* of the projector. Individuals vary greatly in their capacity to use this technique, likewise in their sensitivity to its reception. On the other hand, a strong tendency to use projective identification for very aggressive purposes seems always to be coupled with an increased vulnerability in the face of its aggressive use by others.

If we understand projective identification in this way, we

27

can recognize that the artist during the creative process, when confronted with the anxieties inherent in the flux of relationships to internal objects, at any moment may be impelled by the pain within him to seek relief through projective identification in the sense Mrs. Klein spoke of as 'excessive', that is, excessive in terms of the sadistic and destructive intent of projecting it into other people, due to the complications of the guilt involved, or excessive in the sense of endangering the on-going nature of his own dynamic process. On the other hand we must recognize that the impulse to communicate through projective identification, plays a central part in the normal relation to external objects in the depressive position, implementing the desire, as Bion has stressed, to be understood by objects in the outside world, especially where they are closely linked with the primal good objects of the inner world. It plays an important role also in the relationship to siblings, embodied in the depressive concern for all the mother's babies. I shall come back to this aspect later. What I want to emphasize at this point is that the social impulse involved in artistic creativity—this includes the exhibiting of creations—derives in the first place from the pressure towards projective identification. In constructing a theory of art we must therefore consider the theoretical possibility of what I will call at this point *good* and *evil* art in terms of the motivation behind, not the basic creative process, but behind the exhibiting of the artistic product. In order to avoid muddle in language later on, to use *good* in this sense would mean that we would, in talking about what is ordinarily spoken of as good or bad art, need to change our terms to *successful* and *unsuccessful* art.

At this point I want to introduce two bits of clinical material from children that illustrate the impulse towards artistic productivity derived from the need to use projective identification. One of them is an example of the need to project a destroyed object, and the other is an example of

28

the need to project a destructive part of the self. The first material is from a little girl who was four at the time. In her analysis she was very much preoccupied with her greedy relationship to the breast, following the birth of a sibling who was being breast-fed. During the session I have in mind, she made out of plasticine a little hot-cross-bun which had many times been recognized as linked with the approaching Easter holiday. As soon as I interpreted to her the connection between this good breast, the hot-cross-bun breast, and the anxiety about my going away at Easter, she began to stab and mutilate the little plasticine bun. In the midst of it she stopped, her whole mood changed from vicious attacking to one of smiling benevolence, and she pointed to the box in which her crayons were kept. This box had, on its outside, pictures of animals. She pointed to one of them and said, 'Oh, what a precious little robin redbreast.' You can perhaps see that she was attempting to project this mutilated breast by presenting it in a hypocritically idealized form for me to take in, as though it were something good and beautiful.

STOKES:

I find your interpretation relevant to a danger in the situation of art. It illumines artefacts we call pretty or prettified in a derogatory sense. In so far as such artefacts may without exaggeration be called nauseating, it is to be explained in the manner you have interpreted the 'precious little robin red-breast', a clear gain for understanding, especially in regard to the sugar-coated product that deceives the Philistines: or is it that they would like art to be thus debased? I think they are trying to share the pleasures of art in the sickly and con-tradictory context of denial.

MELTZER:

The experience of nausea, as a mental or physical reaction, illustrates the concreteness with which projective identification works. The second bit of material is derived from a five-year-old boy who in the transference situation, following the weekend, was extremely preoccupied with my children at home and expressed his attacks upon them, representing the attacks on the babies inside the mother's body, by taking the crayons out of his box and breaking the points off. He crushed up these points, verbalizing his vicious attacks on these babies and mashing them up, saying he was making faeces out of them.

At this point the viciousness of his demeanour changed. There was first a moment of anxiety, and then he began to smile, became rather elated, and went over to the tap. He got a little water which he poured on the table, and stirred the bits of crayons which are a type that tends to dissolve in water, making a water colour.

After he had mixed the water and the colours, smiling, and in somewhat of a manic way, he went to his drawer and took out a block of wood and dipped this into the coloured mixture, which was now muddy brown. He then went over to the wall and verbalized that he was printing pictures. Each time he made a muddy smear on the wall he would stand back and admire it, confabulating to it that it was a picture of gates, that it was a picture of trees, there were houses and so forth.

I think that you can see what had happened in this play. During his symbolic attacks on my children, very concrete mutilation was being done to his internal mother's babies. He had suddenly become confronted with an excessively painful situation inside himself, particularly the painful responsibility of depressive feelings connected with the attack, as I knew from previous material. In his exhibiting the process of turning these faeces, derived from attacks on the babies, into paints and then into paintings that I was expected to admire, he was inviting me, by demonstrating the process, to relish, and thereby to wish to emulate, the omnipotence of his creativity. By this means also, of course, he meant to project into me that part of himself that tortured mother by making her watch her babies being killed.

STOKES:

A connection between faeces and paints, between the omnipotent use of faeces and of paint, has often been remarked. You suggest one way that the artist may be rid of his faeces in so far as they contain something bad, while at the same time they provide the means of omnipotence, and even sometimes of good communication.

MELTZER:

Yes; it illustrates the point I referred to earlier when I said that Mrs. Klein had shown that only by knowing the genesis of an object can we be certain of its value. This is perhaps one reason why retrospective shows of an artist's painting are more convincing and reassuring than a single example of his work.

Having now discussed projective identification in both its destructive aspect, and its constructive aspects as an instrument for communication of a primitive and concrete sort, I think we are in a position to examine the psychology of the person who views art. (Of course we are not restricting ourselves to the viewing of visual art only.) I am talking about people who view art as an important, and perhaps even central, part of their inner-life processes. I am therefore excluding the people who view art from more peripheral motivations. It will perhaps be useful to indicate that, in so far as contemplating art is a form of intercourse between viewer and artist, it has an exact parallel in the sexual relationships between individuals. We would want to distinguish here between events in which sexual relationships are casual regarding choice of partner, being in this sense a direct extension of the masturbation process. (By this I don't mean

31

to imply necessarily that it is an extremely harmful or sadistic matter.) In contrast, there are those events of sexual intercourse in which contact with the other person's inner world is central. Here, of course, we would have to distinguish between acts of love and acts of sadism, again in the latter case not necessarily implying that these acts of sadism would have to be carried out in objectively perverse ways. In acts of love we know very well that processes both of projecting love and good objects, as well as of introjecting from the love-partner, are going on. In a similar way, in a destructive intercourse the projecting of bad parts of the self and of the destroyed objects, as well as the masochistic submission of one's self to this form of abuse are enacted. There is a parallel, then, in the intercourse between the artist and the viewer: the artistic production itself is a very concrete representation of what is transported. I think that the viewer we have in mind is not at all at play: while his social relationship to his companions may be part of his play life, towards art he is *at work*, exposing himself to a situation of intensely primitive (oral) introjection through his eyes or ears or sense of touch. That is, he enters a gallery with the aim of carrying out an infantile introjection, with the hope, in its constructive aspects, of obtaining something in the nature of a reconstructed object. Conversely, in a masochistic sense, a viewer may be going to expose himself to the experience of having projected into him a very destroyed object or a very bad part of the self of the artist. This aspect of masochism I have discussed a bit in my paper on Tyranny.

I would like to illustrate this with clinical material from the same little boy that I've spoken of in regard to the printing on the wall. At a point in his treatment when he was in extremely close touch with me as a good mother who was feeding him the analysis, he was standing by the table, leaning against me, with his thumb in mouth, after having asked me to draw for him a diagram of the analysis and the sessions he would be having until Christmas. During the time he was leaning against me, he was looking at the wall opposite and said, 'Oh, it's so shiny, like a television screen!' And he said, 'Oh, I can see fishes swimming around.' At this point he took his thumb out of his mouth and commented that it was quite shiny too, that he could see in it the reflection of the light bulb that was over my head. He then very carefully, keeping his eye on this shiny spot on his thumb, put it back in his mouth and said, 'I've got it.' What I want to bring out in this material is that this little boy was having an intense experience of sucking on the breast, and you can see that sucking on the breast was accompanied by a particularly vivid experience of feeling able to look inside the mummy's body and to see all her little fish-babies restored, swimming about—it is implied—quite happily free from his usual attacking impulses. That is the kind of breast and breast-mother he felt himself to be introjecting at this point, represented by the shiny spot reflecting the light bulb that he put into his mouth and sucked upon. I am suggesting to you that the viewing of art is an expression particularly linked to this component of the breast situation, that is, the feeling of looking and listening to the events going on inside the mother, of seeing either the intactness of her inner world, or conversely, of seeing the destruction that has been wrought there. It means an experience of allowing, in the first case, the introjecting of this goodness and intactness and, in the second case, exposing oneself to having destruction projected into one.

STOKES:

I think you could say that because an evocation of the breast relationship and of the relationship to the mother herself are built into formal presentation as a perennial basis, we are induced, far more strongly than we would otherwise be, to contemplate the detailed reflections of the processes of the inner life that a work of art may contain.

What you have said about the oral introjection performed by the viewer points particularly to the enveloping action of a work of art and to the breast relationship from which it derives. The work of art is basically a reconstruction not only of the whole and independent object but of the part-object, the beneficent breast. I refer once more to the general, the formal, value rather than to the impact, thereby magnified, of a subject-matter that may be negative, that may invite, as you suggest a masochistic state of mind. I would only add, in part; that even in such a case the post-depressive co-ordination altogether necessary, we are agreed, to the creating of art, will have been affirmed, transmitted, however indirectly. To put it another way; when a discernment of inner states, however horrific, however dispensable by means of a sadistic projection, is stabilized in terms of aesthetic oppositions and balances and other aspects of form, some coordination, some bringing together, will have occurred at the expense of denial; and this bringing together will have required, at the fount, the shadow of a reconstructed whole-object and part-object whose presence can at least be glimpsed in the very existence of an aesthetic result. Thus, a painting that represents violence, disintegration, provided it be a good painting, of the full calibre of art, should remain not at all unpleasant to live with, day in day out. Earlier on, you have distinguished between 'the creativity, the projection of it' and 'the exhibiting of the artistic product.' I am not so willing to separate as entirely as you do for some instances, all the motivations in these two activities.

To avoid misunderstanding, I think we should remark that the fact that many people are disgusted or outraged by a new departure in art, does not necessarily have a predominant bearing on the intentions, conscious or otherwise, of the artist. In my paper I discussed the dislike of art from the point of view of the fear aroused by so vivid a comment upon

34

psychical reality. Maybe, though, this is important in putting the artist on his mettle.

As to sexual intercourse as a process identical in its method with relationship to the art-object, while endorsing the interchanges between viewer and picture that you suggest, I would like to add that the relationship exists, as does the parallel, only because of the essential otherness, the character of self-subsistent entity, the complement to the breast relationship, that has been created.

MELTZER:
We are agreed that the successful work of art is compelling; it induces a process in us, an experience whereby the viewer's integration is called upon in the depressive position to restrain his attacking impulses, for the sake of a good introjection; it means allowing the good object to make a good kind of projection into one's inner world. It requires judgement to distinguish the good from the bad processes of sadism in the artist and masochism in himself, the viewer. I think it follows, therefore, that the experience of viewing art can be extremely taxing and extremely hazardous, but that the artworld, as an institution within our culture, provides a medium for people to carry out this introjective process in an atmosphere of relative external safety, corresponding to the safety of the little infant in the relative restraint of the mother's arms. When one walks into an art gallery, one is surrounded by other people and there are guards and so on; all this constitutes a continual external support to one's internal safeguards against attacking the pieces of art that are exhibited there. Similarly at a concert. It is well known that, in contrast to this safe viewing of art, at times of revolution or warfare, pillaging includes a wholesale destruction of everything of artistic value. There are instances when people of extremely unbalanced mental state have attacked priceless works of art in galleries.

35

I want now to discuss the implications as regards the social motivation in the artist for producing and exhibiting good works of art. I presume that this social motivation is present from the beginning of his artistic development but that it becomes stronger and stronger as his maturity as an artist is achieved, maturity not only of mastery over his materials but particularly of the sense of stabilization through his artistic activity and other processes in his social and internal life, of his relationship to his own primal good objects in his inner world. I have said earlier that it is necessary for a theoretical approach to recognize the possibility of evil motivation in the exhibiting of art, that is, either as a means of projecting the persecutory or depressive anxieties connected with destroyed objects into viewers or, worse, as a means of corrupting and attacking their internal relationships. But I have also stressed that the motivation for exhibiting good works of art is derived from two sources: first of all from the desire to be understood and appreciated by others, as an important element for reinforcing the capacity to carry on with painful struggle toward the depressive position; and second, I have implied that there comes a point of stabilization in the inner world when that element of the depressive position that has to do with feelings of concern for 'all the mother's babies' becomes very dominant. At this point, I believe, the impulse to exhibit works of art, representing the artist's progress in working through his depressive conflicts, begins to take a form that could rightly be called the impulse to *sermonize*. In this sense every work of art, from such a period of an artist's life, has the function of a *sermon to siblings*, a sermon which is not only intended to show what has been accomplished by this brother but is also intended to project into the siblings both the restored object as well as to project those capacities for the bearing of depressive pains which have been achieved by the artist in his own development. Seen from the spectator's angle, the viewing, and the yearning to view, the work of

36

masters would not only derive from the relationship to the product of art as representing the mother's body and the contents of her body; it also represents the relationship to the artist as an older sibling from whom this kind of encouragement and help in achieving a sufficient devotion and reverence for the parent is sought.

STOKES:

You have now carried further your contribution on the role of projective identification. It brings me a feeling of light, first in regard to a matter that has been of particular importance. Things made by man please and depress the aesthete through a mode far more intimate than in his contemplation of Nature. You explain it by introducing the projective identifications of which the viewer of art is the recipient. I wish there had been the occasion for you to re-introduce here from your Tyranny paper your conception of the smugness remaining in the projector of evil, and that you had brought it to bear in connection with a remark you made to me about the effect on us of much Victorian architecture.

As to sermonizing to siblings, I cannot refrain from mentioning that I found long ago that I could provide no other word than 'brotherliness' to denote an interplay of equal, non-emphatic, forms in some of the greatest painting.

In applying psycho-analysis to the social value of art, to the manner of communication and to the role it plays in the calculations and satisfactions of the artist himself, you make a new beginning. It is from your angle, I think, that what appears to be the slavery of the artist will be most fruitfully approached, an aspect, I have pointed out elsewhere, entirely ignored by psycho-analysis. I mean the subjection of the artist to his time, and therefore to the art of his time, inasmuch as art must reflect typical concatenations of experience, of endeavour, in the milieu in which the artist and his public live; otherwise the artist's achievement of form seems to be nearly always without urgency or power. This cultural expression of significant dispositions both perennial and topical (underlying the creation of significant form) that may completely change the emotional bent, as well as the style, of art, will have entailed a novel psychical emphasis. Since we aesthetes are inclined to agree that the creator's prime social task is to help his siblings with their conflicts in a contemporary setting, identifying stress and the resolving of it with accentuations appropriate to a particular environment, just as each individual on his own is bound to do; since the artist's attainment of aesthetic value is understood to be inseparable from what is both subservience and leadership, we realize at once the penetration of your approach.

I fear that this may sound as if I thought a painter's work must include sociological comment. Of course it is not so. He is concerned with value in the inside and outside world, the value of landscape, say, to himself and to his contemporaries, a value that sometimes entails resuscitation of a discarded aesthetic tradition as he looks with new eyes, conditioned by current ideas, not only at Nature but at the art of the past. This application of the inner world to outside situations accords with the sensuous condition of art and especially with some degree of naturalism.

MELTZER:

I believe that the question you are raising now is one we must attempt to deal with if this present paper is to make a contribution, for, as I have said to you privately, all that we have been discussing up to this point has been either stated or adumbrated by yourself and Dr. Segal. Because of the concreteness of the splitting within the early ego, during the reintegration process of the depressive position the different fragments of the self hold a relationship to one another as siblings. It is characteristic, as seen in the analytic process, that the reappearance of a formerly widely-split-off part of

38

the self, and its renewed availability for integration within
the sphere of the primal good objects, are experienced by
the already-integrated parts of the self as a 'new baby'
situation. The resistance to the admission of this little stranger
to the family of the integrated self derives from the spectrum
of anxieties and jealousies characteristic of the birth of a
sibling. But against these resistances is balanced the pull of
the good objects, the determination of the parent figures to
nurture *all* their children, regardless of qualities, hopeful of
enriching the impoverished, and pacifying the rabid.

Such is the painful struggle in psychical reality towards
integration of the split-off parts of the self and towards
embracing *all the mother's and father's babies*. Progress in
psychical reality is accompanied by modifications in attitudes
and behaviour in external reality. Idealization of the in-
group, and its corresponding paranoia, diminish. Guilt-laden
feelings of responsibility, mixed always with contempt, give
way to more genuine concern and respect for the potentialities
of others.

But where progress is considerable—and I think this is
often experienced by people in analysis—a very painful
disequilibrium comes to pass, where the internal sibling-
parts of the self improve, and the security and happiness of
the primal good objects correspondingly improve, far in
excess of what can be seen to be going on between siblings
and mother earth in the external world. Also it becomes
evident, as processes of reparation are more firmly established
in psychical reality, that its corresponding process in the
external world is very partial, limited by the frailty of the
human body and its limited power of rejuvenation, extra-
polating to zero at death. Further, the laws of psychical reality
differ considerably from the laws of external reality where
non-human agencies, structuralized as 'fate', play with human
affairs, ten tragedies to every farce.

The agonizing problem thus becomes: How to live with a

relatively harmonious inner world enriched by the bounty and beauty of one's good objects, in an outside world that mirrors its beauty but not its harmony, *about which one can no longer remain unconcerned.* This, I suggest, is the task from which the mature, exhibiting artist does not flee, but, to borrow Hanna Segal's words, with his 'cautionary tales', he sets about 'repairing the whole world.' It implies that an artist must sermonize his siblings as they exist *at that moment*: that the formal and emotive configuration of his works must be derived not only from the influence exerted upon him by his culture and fellow artists, but also by the force of his *concern* with the present and future of the whole world. In order to grasp the courage that this requires of such an artist, it is necessary to realize that every act of violence which he sees go unpunished and, above all, smugly unrepented, every cruel stroke of fate in the external world, threatens his internal harmony because of the pain and rage stirred. Thus, concern for the outside world increases the temptation to renew the old splitting and projection of bad parts of the self. The pull of the monastery becomes tremendous as a bulwark against the danger of regression.

STOKES:
Perhaps another time we shall construct our version of the artist as hero, with comment upon the growing cult that helps to inspire the present furore for art, especially the acclaim of Gauguin and Van Gogh.

You leave it to me to take up your distinction of good and evil art in the sense that a work of art is either predominantly reassuring or corrupting to its audience, as opposed to good and bad art aesthetically considered. As you know, while I agree with your formulation of reassuring and corruptive projective identifications ceaselessly transmitted through art—evaluatory criticism is inseparable from acts of correct appreciation—I trust more in the fact that a projection cannot be regarded as art unless some degree of an integrative blend of emotion, typical of the depressive position as you have defined it, shall thereby be communicated. Provided that it is deeply understood, I cannot view any true work of art to be predominantly corrupting in its many aftermaths. Perhaps I am the more ready to value very greatly what you have said about the social importance of projective identification since I have already considered other primitive mechanisms, though subject to the depressive position, to be embodied in art.

You emphasize you are concerned only with the social aspect, not with the aesthetic aspect on which we are agreed. But consider for a moment what Mario Praz has called in his famous book of that name, *The Romantic Agony*, consider the nineteenth century intertwining themes of satanism, sadism, masochism, homosexuality, of Medusa, Salome and the Gioconda smile, of the ruthless and fatal woman, *La Belle Dame sans Merci*, common to Flaubert and to the pre-Raphaelites, or of the Faustian Byronic man; an ethos to frame the savagery of Delacroix, the sudden ambivalence of Berlioz, the perversity of Baudelaire, great artists who were impelled to magnify at arm's length that which, in themselves as in the world, was untoward. By means of uneasy juxtapositions through their art, of beauty and despair or squalor, they sustained acrid versions of the integrative process. On the other hand, the celebrations of sadism— De Sade himself is the key, said Sainte-Beuve, to the literature of that time—and of masochism in which so many artists joined, did not do them, not to speak of their public, much good. It seems that self-destruction in some cases was the mode of liberation from cruel Victorian smugness. The first theme of all was the one of masochism. We need to integrate Swinburne's obsession with flagellation not only with his public school experiences but, more widely, with the cruelly smug Victorian culture to which he truthfully responded,

41

in so far as his obsession inspired very considerable poems; we need to bring into relation with the milieu what Praz described as 'the lustful pleasure in contamination' that characterized so many romantics and decadents; Baudelaire's confessed aim of seeking beauty in evil; Lautréamont's concentration upon evil to make, as he felt, the reader desire good. As well as a dire creative synthesis often of the utmost beauty and courage, in all such cases one is likely as well to detect a straightforward element of bad projective identification.

A considerable amount of the romantic agony survives today. A mitigation, I feel, is due to Freud, though he has inspired further manifestations. Seen from the angle of art, Freud largely took over from artists the mere ventilation of specific perversions. It is well worth mentioning that a scientific discovery about the psyche could somewhat modify the central position of an artistic subject-matter. It shows in this case that, unlike the perennial reaching after violence in newspaper, popular novel and film, on which so many people have the necessity to feed, sensationalism in art includes as well an attempt at description, at understanding, hence at integration. I am inclined to think that artists, more than any other class perhaps, tend to find themselves unresponsive to daily sensationalism not widely symbolic, owing to the gratuitous quality, owing to a lack of reality or connection. It is significant, however, that it should be generally felt that art alone justifies a presentation of what otherwise would be unacceptable; art is felt to be a constructive if desperate or daring comment, though the artist may also be projecting into us the aggression by which he and his objects are threatened. What you have said about the depressive devotion to truth and the connection with beauty, is most relevant here. But if, in this extravagant process, we, as spectators, find ourselves to be losers, then we say that those particular paintings are no good; no good, as far as a simple judge-

42

ment of acceptance or dismissal is concerned, in your sense and in an aesthetic sense as well, since there is no aesthetic value without co-ordination, or, put negatively, without an overall lack of gratuitousness. Of course people will vary in their estimations of what is gratuitous: the more experienced in art usually find the less experienced to be timid, narrow about the channels through which they gain a positive meaning: similarly—at any rate to some extent—psychoanalysts may find others to be incorrigibly blind to the pathetic, even, at times, constructive, aspects of delinquency. It is remarkable, surely, that though cultural situations alter, no considerable achievement in art ceases to have relevance. The urgency of bringing together, of making one thing out of what is diverse, remains unique just because the material varies yet continues to give echo, to make itself felt and thereby to encourage us, even in those instances where we have reason to deplore emotional ingredients on display.

MELTZER:
This view of the artist, that he mobilizes powerful psychological equipment and that he exerts a great influence on his culture seems tacitly accepted; it is evidenced by the reverence (dead) artists receive, by local and national pride based on their creativity. But of course the more open attitude toward (living) artists is very different. Where grudging admiration is given to their craftsmanship, their characters are condemned: where the social and political importance of their work is not sneered at as the mere embellishment of history, the state or patrons may attempt to exploit and control them: where they are not beggared and neglected, they are treated as pets or *enfants terribles*. To sum it up psycho-analytically, until they become 'masters' they are treated as new babies at the breast, by a world full of siblings who, while deriving hope from the new baby's existence and performance, cannot control their envy and jealousy.

43

Now, the aspects of psychical reality acted out through the socio-*economic* structure of society, are in part related psycho-analytically with the impulses to master and exploit the breasts and body of the bad, deserting and begrudging mother, fickle and selective in the granting of her favours, united to the powerful and punitive father. Flux in these aspects of group life, with ever-accelerating tempo, is constantly induced by technological advance (note, I speak of the application of knowledge, not of advances in knowledge itself, i.e. of technology, not of science). The phantasy of plundering this bad mother's body, of tyrannizing over her inner babies, is the driving force, I believe, behind economic aggression.

Juxtaposed to this unstable situation, constantly stirred by technological advance, there exists the socio-*aesthetic* life of people, presided over by the art-world. Here the internal reality of the good, or, as you point out, often idealized mother and her breasts, united to the good, creative and reparative father and his penis, find expression, reminding the children of the bounty of life and the relative insignificance of the differences in nature's gifts when compared with the great expanse of biological equality in the human life-cycle. The art-world is the institutionalization of the social forces towards integration. Earlier I have spoken, for the purpose of exemplification, of the viewing of art as if it were something limited to museums, concert halls and libraries. In fact the art-world monopolizes expression of the beauty and goodness of psychical reality, the craving for which no riches of external nature can gratify. In nature we can find reflected the beauty we already contain. But art helps us to regain what we have lost.

New References

BION, W. R. *Thinking* (unpublished).
KLEIN, M. *Envy and Gratitude* (London, 1957).
MELTZER, D. *The Interpretation of Tyranny* (unpublished).
PRAZ, M. *The Romantic Agony* (London, 1933).

TOWARDS THE SOCIAL BASIS OF ART

New Reference

III. THE ART OF TURNER
1775–1851

III. The Art of Turner (1775-1851)

Art opposes self-concealment; painting should reveal its student. Nudity, an absolute achieved so often in an instant without rebuff, furnishes no reference to the endless mind. On the contrary, great artists deepen the search in themselves, pierce for a moment a hardly won aesthetic integration in order to disclose and to re-align the detail of which it was fashioned. This further self cannot fructify into masterpieces except through the manner of uncovering more art within the art that the painter, and other painters, have already achieved. Subject to patronage, to social needs, the Old Master had to provide *from his beginning* a stiff apparel of stable co-ordination. Did he then probe concomitantly the self and its art, he sometimes introduced less polished, more weighty, 'sermons to siblings'. Though ostensibly, in the final phases of Rembrandt and Turner, the artist was working more to please himself alone, the exploration of his art cannot be removed from the desire to communicate by means of it.

But what if there is no achievement to explore but only the self and art in general? A modern student's rather noisy searching of his canvas for a dynamic aspect of himself is by no means the consequence of intensifying a compulsion that was already implicit within his work, since he is just starting to paint. He seeks a mode for what psycho-analysts call 'acting out', of living upon the canvas in terms of brush and paint and strength of arm. This is not a fair description since his activities are symbolic: I use the expression, 'acting out', because although the process of sublimation, upon which art depends, is present, it can be minimized in the reckoning. With serious, perhaps painful, attention the student searches the face of the canvas for what he supposes to be barely hidden within himself. At the same time he may regard the physical act of painting as if it were a therapy applied to objects, just as the right tune in the right ambience seems to agitate surroundings towards a dynamic concord. Communication, the learning of means of communication, are at a discount. Since we are rich in photographs and in museums, poor in cultural stability and settled style, and even of patrons' commands, we fragment the interwoven values of art, tend to use one piece to mirror a sum of compulsions. In the past, on the other hand, a narrowly compulsive element would encounter from the beginning, would emerge, perhaps only finally to overlay, a hundred matters other than the canvas and the paints. That process encouraged aesthetic power, especially the enveloping factor in form, since a hoard of self-sufficient experiences and achievements would therein be embraced. The modern tendency inclines towards a series that together, and only together, as a whole exhibition, can rival the impact of a single masterpiece.

There is a long history of indistinctness in Turner's art, connected throughout with what I have called an embracing or enveloping quality, not least of the spectator with the picture. The power grew in Turner of isolating the visionary effectiveness that belongs to a passing event of light: it entailed some loss of definition in the interest of emphasis upon an overall quality. To one who complained, Turner is said to have replied: 'Indistinctness is my forte'. I shall attempt interpretation of a narrow compulsion that I attribute to a predominant aspect of his embracing effects: my aim will be to suggest how minor this theme would probably have proved had it been abstracted from the lengthy apprenticeship of its intrusion, had it not been long attendant upon contrasting achievements in picture-making. His supremacy lies not in his compulsions but in the links established for them, subsidiary yet vastly enriching. It is a matter of degree, for otherwise it is the same with every artist. Our interest today in aesthetic directness, though in many senses estimable, in another can be not a little vulgar. Aesthetic directness, so far from always enjoying a lack of limitation, may itself be inhibited by an expressiveness that casts away the many links for a compulsion, that avoids contrast, the means of sublimation as well as material for integration. But we cannot summon at a wish what I have called subsidiary and enriching aims: should they be potential, however, understanding will encourage their presence.

Turner's visions founded on Rome and Venice developed gradually over many years. When he first went to Italy he had concentrated on topographical drawings and sketches, no less than 1500 or so in probably little over two months, of Rome, Naples and the surroundings. The habit of drawing must have asserted itself every day, and often all day. One reason why in the sketch-books there are so many drawings of Dover Castle and the coast, will have been due to his waits there for the continental packet. Do we have comparable disciplines? Moreover his memory for natural effect was no less fully rehearsed than his power to observe it.

We shall find that the accustomed objects of his art, buildings among foliage, trees, mountains, ships, eventually shared their qualities with their media, buildings with the sky, ships with the sea and vice versa: finally, sky and water were equated with the paint itself even for large works: the equation had long been brought about for some drawings and sketches, including oil sketches. In a word, the homogeneous effect we admire so much, supervened upon a thousand studies amassed from many kinds of objects under the aegis of contemporary styles for picture-making and of a naturalistic bent that was never lost: the artist with the mood of nature were first established by the paint and, in the end,

51

as the paint, a contemporary effect that seems far less comfortable as a first endeavour. The chief of all painting problems is here: the journeyman starts at the point where a supreme master lay down the brush, not one master but many; many more today than at any time before.

A first reference should be to the social determinant of Turner's art, the studies to provide whatever patrons would admire and, as the result of unceasing industry, to earn a good living. The early topographical watercolours and others from which engravings were made—the first was published when he was just nineteen—depended for their value, of course, upon the sentiment infusing their fact, upon the element of communicated 'truth', the theme ever-present in art that Dr. Meltzer brought into relation with care and love for the object conceived in the depressive or post-depressive position. Viewed as a 'sermon to siblings', visual art seeks to reflect and embody some of the needs or tensions of a society, and of the artist's inner world, *vis-à-vis* Nature, in terms of the outside world. The painter is he whose inner world, everywhere intertwined with the outer, will be projected in such a way as to communicate to his fellows a freshness of feeling about objects; ultimately, though often most superficially, the feeling of being more at home in a grown-up world. We have seen that the scale of aesthetic integration will vary with conditions of culture and of preceding art. If we believe in the truth for him of what Turner wrote in a margin of Opie's lectures, from the viewpoint of today we shall consider that he was extremely fortunate regarding the historical context. . . . 'every look at Nature is a refinement upon art', he wrote: and he continues by saying he conceives the painter as 'admiring Nature by the power and practicability of his Art, and judging of his Art by the perceptions drawn from Nature'. (As to Art, it has been said that the last ten years of the eighteenth century, the time of Turner's youth, was the best there had yet been in London

for students of post-Renaissance European painting, due
largely to big sales following the French Revolution.)

The study of Turner, then, is a robust yet romantic subject:
part of the attraction is his silence, the devotion to his work
from the early morning; each year for many years the tours
that uncovered the rewarding aspects of the English scene
at a period when many English towns and villages were
astonishingly beautiful, at a moment of poignant beauty
inasmuch as the threat of great changes was sometimes
implicit: at a period when the smaller country-seat domains
were multiplying in number and optimism; when the achievements of Trafalgar and Copenhagen fortified ordinary pride.
It is the countryside as we still want it to be; consequently,
in spite of what I have said about the uniqueness of the
moment of any art, we do not often think of Turner as an
eighteenth century or a Regency or an early Victorian figure.
His vein of romantic mastery was embodied also in the
prescient, was somewhat committed, Kenneth Clark has
pointed out, even to the baby triumphs of a growing mechani-
cal age. With the vigour and cockiness of small stature he
embraced the huge variety of a scene as we would have it
not altogether nostalgically, because we cannot altogether
believe that it no longer exists: a gleam from what remains
reconstitutes an unaltered conviction about the countryside,
reinforced especially by Turner's panoramas of the coast
from out at sea or from near the beach where, often, there has
been no change. On the other hand the early sea-pieces, and
views of shipping that he discerned with a naval eye, are
among the more 'dated' of his works.

Turner's encircling contemplation was for long closely
tied, except in sketches, to the adjunct of several old pictorial
traditions, particularly the Dutch. An astonishing factor in
his development was the direct rivalry with Claude to which
he felt himself constrained; it is only emphasized by his
preference for Punic rather than for the Roman and Grecian

heroes. For a long time, perhaps to the end, Turner chose to regard *Dido building Carthage* (exhib: 1815) as his *chef d'œuvre*. Involved today with pictorial 'break-through', we are astonished not so much that Sir George Beaumont objected to them as that it was apt enough, in spite of their incipient romantic unity, for him to judge Turner's earlier oil paintings in terms of Cuyp, Ruysdael, Claude, artists who had been dead for more than a hundred years. Due to a variety and development that spans such distance, Turner contrived connections that we find reassuring. Moreover, as I have said, he made out of many-sidedness more powerful ammunition for very personal bents or compulsions: incorporated thus with perennial psychical requirements, they furnish most important lessons to us his siblings. Of course the message of truth in Turner's work was not at all the one of a sociological survey. His nightmares are by no means specific to that terrible age. He gives us what he, as an artist, felt, but rarely what others, figuring in his paintings, might be feeling. Of this, we shall realize, he was almost incapable. Not that he did not often admit its propriety on a small and crowded scale, sometimes with passable result, for instance *The Shipwreck* (exhibited 1805).

But before considering the more extreme aspects of the Turner subject, we must take some cognizance of tension in the aesthetic situation. What we can view as a spanning— by Girtin as by Turner—became a struggle, a tension seen in the rival advocacies of light and darker paintings, largely as a result of the influence upon oil painting of the effects and technical inventions in watercolour. Turner was accused most variously of being hesitant, of sacrificing the precept of art to the vulgarities of nature, of vagueness as of brittleness and, even as early as 1798 when he was twenty-three, of a mannered approach.

Crabb Robinson entered in his diary for May 7th, 1825: 'Went to the Exhibition, with the advantage of having my

54

attention drawn to the best pictures which, for the most part, equalled my expectations. Turner, R.A., has a magnificent view of Dieppe. If he will invent an atmosphere, and a play of colours all his own, why will he not assume a romantic name (for his pictures)? No one could find fault with a garden of Armida, or even of Eden, so painted. But we know Dieppe, in the north of France, and can't easily clothe it in such faery hues. I can understand why such artists as Constable and Collins are preferred.' It seems that Turner's effects of light and atmosphere did not appear to correspond with their natural phenomena because the eye of the cultured spectator was still viewing Nature, in front of pictures at least, through the glass of an older art. On the other hand, Crabb Robinson perceives that Turner's overall paintings of light and atmosphere could pass as his version of acceptable pictorial manipulations that belonged especially to the eighteenth century. Even in many of his earlier historical paintings that aped the past, or were meant to rival it, mythological incident took but a small place, not only in area as in Claudes, but in regard to the mood of a landscape or of a meteorological happening. A more truthful, because more transitory, natural effect was the vehicle in his hands of an emotion that was less restrained, yet without the entire loss, all the same, of the feeling for a contrived magnitude in virtue of which we at once recognize a classical composition. The presence in sketch book numbered 90 in the Turner Bequest of contiguous studies, suggest for a few instances a possibility that the conceiving of a classical composition may have included its projection upon familiar Thames-side scenes, particularly the pile of Windsor Castle. It would be in tune with Turner's literary orientation, powerful to the end, from the eighteenth-century sublimities of Thomson. At that time Turner was living in Sion Ferry House, Isleworth. A few years before he had painted many oil sketches on the Thames direct from nature, a rare procedure for him, in-

E   55

frequent in the case of watercolours as opposed to pencil drawings. I feel that he was able later to conjoin the London Thames as such with Venice as such. I must repeat that the greatness of Turner, and indeed the originality, was first of all the product of the diversities he linked as he drew upon much experience. I shall soon suggest that a savage compulsion dramatized his power of linking, absorbed into homogeneous effects the varieties of connectiveness. The variety of homogeneous effect is itself astounding. Applied to Turner's painting, the adjective, 'homogeneous', suggests very late brilliant, light-toned canvases with hardly a perpendicular feature, or else a whirlpool envelopment by fire, flood, incipient in all his landscape styles except the first and in some degree, the last. Yet at the very time of his enlargement of a direct, panchromatic oil technique in the 1830s, he was still painting grey sea paintings sometimes of limpid scenes, one of his versions of the Dutch tradition. These, it appears to me, though undemonstrative, no less than the all-devouring dramas hot or cold, prefigure the unified substance of the later canvases whose breadth has needed dual lineage. Thus, Turner's application was wide. He gained some victories even in the field of calm, contemplative genre (*Blacksmith's Shop*, exhib. 1807, culminating in *Frosty Morning*, exhib. 1813): nor can one forget, though far less successful, what may be called (cf. Rothenstein & Butlin) the Rembrandt and Watteau figure compositions of the 1820s.

Doubtless attracted by Watteau's colour as by Stothard's, Turner was no more suited to emulate rococo elements than in verses his much-beloved Thomson, poet of the picture-like or picturesque. A measure of incongruity, it seems, added fuel to his ambition: what grew in him, what he fostered, consorted ill in some respects with the physical impression he made, with a rusted, hard-bitten (by persecutory fears) man of business; yet he joined them, in his art not least a

56

sometimes stilted version of eighteenth-century sublimity
with the inordinate ranging of romantic verve.

Venice was part of his inheritance, particularly the Venice
of Canaletto. His three visits probably amounted in all to
about six weeks: the first, on the journey to Rome in 1819
when he made some detailed topographical drawings and
many sketches, will have subsequently intensified a myth-
ology of conflagration and reflection. But whereas, hitherto,
he had romanticized the strength of building, architecture
in some very late Venetian paintings serves no more than as a
grandiloquent sail amid the suffusion of sea with sky, a
medium for the riding of blanched or darkened boats. I
think Turner gained confidence for a lengthy elucidation of
light from his encounter in 1802 with the Old Masters at the
Louvre. The criticism written in his sketch-book is concerned
almost entirely with falsity of light effect and poverty of
colour combinations. He was to dissolve the kind of chiaroscuro that dramatizes the world's actuality, in favour of a
diffused light that took actuality to itself, even in finished
drawings, particularly those he made for their engraving
where an equality of effect often overrides most subtly,
without undermining, the strong chiaroscuro and sturdy
relief, even though the initial terms to be unified within the
envelope were alternations of the topographical or romantic
classical stones, the buildings he had so long studied, towering
stone, so often towering above, offset by the dark density of
foliage. Precipitous building led to the appalling paths of
tossed sea, to mountains and cloud and to towering effects of
light. The first link between early and late Turner is the one
between the mutual enhancement of textures to which he
was very sensitive, and of those of colour or light: in painting,
texture and colour sensations can be very close. To my mind
Turner's perceptiveness for building—the unreliable Thornbury reports Mr. Trimmer the younger as having heard
Turner wish that he had been an architect—and for the sense

57

of suffusion in ordered stone with water that much Italianate art had diversified on the example of Venice and of Rome, inspire the slabs of iridescent colour we think of when we call to mind his late works, no less dynamic in themselves than the imaginative drama and sense of doom and other obvious instruments by which he engineers an overall effect of a majesty to approach the gravity and balance attained by earlier Masters. His poetic discernment first fed upon, then diversified as the pictorial instrument, the close enhancements of texture or of colour, and so of shape.

If the deepest aim was transcendent, Turner employed for it his vast experience of measure. There is small appearance of the arbitrary in his drifts of mountain, sea and sky: they formulate an erratic architecture or a superb natural habitat, no less than an irresistible phenomenon; soft and tenuous, warmed as well as cold. It was as if catastrophes were carvings on the sky: they stem from the delicate use of the pencil in thousands of drawings, slight touches to enrich the paper as if it were a volume invoked by this touch, remarkable not only for delicacy but for selectiveness, even in so early an architectural drawing as the sketch of Stamford, Lincolnshire, of 1797. Unity of treatment is matched by that of feeling: what is grasped from the subject is accorded with the projected strain of feeling that encompasses and adjusts each detail with another. Turner not only thought of himself as a poetic painter but attempted poetry, at times to introduce his pictures. He may have intended to preface the *Southern Coast* series of engravings with a long narrative poem. His use of words became stiff, repetitious, very confused; so also, very often, the delineation of people in his landscapes.

His growing love of overall effect without loss to the representation of endless distance, the palpability for many ripe works of the picture plane, prime overall unit, suggest some parallel with our own preoccupations: many drawings, often of the earlier years, prefigure in this respect late Turner oil painting. For instance the 'Salisbury' sketch-book of about 1800 (T.B.49) has two scribbles of sunset, clouds and water, integrated as one mass: another early instance (1802) is a wonderful little drawing—the Finberg catalogue says probably of Brienz—made up of abbreviated hooked strokes (T.B.77). The minuscule mosaic of angularity, the richness in the poverty, suggest Klee to us. Much earlier, in 1795 when Turner was twenty, he could achieve a not dissimilar compositional effect of the greatest delicacy, such as the twin drawings of two mounted figures descending a hill-side path near the sea (T.B. 25). Other drawings conjure up Cézanne: even in many grand paintings some values of the sketch are obstinately maintained. Although there is evidence that Turner would not allow rough pencil sketches to be glimpsed, he seems to have had more faith in his handling than had Constable in his, an artist, we may suspect, who was on less good terms with himself. Even the technique in some last oils where calligraphy overlays an unbroken cake of paint, is foreshadowed by very delicate pencil drawings on paper prepared with wash rubbed out for the lights, such as in the beautiful 'Dunbar' sketch-book of 1801 (T.B. 54) or the 1802 'Schaffhausen' folio set (T.B. 79) or, better still, the radiant drawings of the 1819 'Tivoli' sketch-book (T.B. 183). On the other hand there are prosaic finished watercolours of the middle period that have very low value, such as *Saltash* in the Lloyd Bequest. Until much later, Turner was still apt to demarcate his work for the public in agreement with the traditional genres.

A price had to be paid for the homogeneous effect, a price on which Turner's critics were agreed; not only that: his flattening of figures and tempering of foreground in the interest of overall effect corresponded to a lack of *inevitable* interest in relief, shown by the playing down of figures as a result of his growing concentration upon the enveloping landscape. We shall find that these attitudes are possibly linked in deeper layers of the mind also. On the other hand, early studies of buildings, hills, and especially rocks, are often very notable for their relief. Turner was a phenomenal draughtsman in several genres, but particularly for choice and disposition of accent and bare space in a finely controlled sea of detail; for a pointilliste employment as a youth, in company with Girtin, of the pencil's point within a pattern of short strokes. His drawings of the figure at the Academy schools were no more than adequate. Some later drawings of the nude are considerably better, but do not obtain high significance. Except in the case of cows and of the early self-portrait in oil, his delineation of faces seems wooden. We cannot discover in Turner's art much affirmative relationship to the whole body, to human beings. They tend to be sticks, or fish that bob or flop or are stuffed. The prejudice is sometimes allowed such freedom, that many figures who should be dignified appear to be rustic, to be approached by the artist with unconcealed because untutored naïvety, though this is in fact very far from the case. To use the psycho-analytic term, they suggest part-objects. (A part-object, it may be recalled, is an organ or function that on the analogy of the first object, the breast, has been split off from an object's other organs and functions: a part-object, therefore, is a concept at a great distance from the one of a whole, separate person for whom, in a regression, it may come to stand).

Turner's chosen relaxation was to fish. (The drawing of young anglers for the *Liber Studiorum* is among his most engaging figure-groups). He saw the feminine in cows but upon human life he tended to bestow a phallic cast. He himself was small, rather Punch-like, deliberate and usually taciturn. (His father, even more Punch-like in appearance, was more talkative). Ruskin found elongated figures, oval elms and flat-topped pines to be typical Turnerian shapes.

Also typical, after 1820, is the curvilinear form of crutch or thigh bone along the side of which, as in the *Palestrina* painting, there runs a narrow vent. Very upright figures, such as the one of the strange *Letter*, may amount to the crutch-shape with attendant valley. They include Phryne at the edge of the huge painting named after her. The many Turner- or Punch-faced people who inelegantly, if wraith-like, throng *Richmond Hill on the Prince Regent's Birthday*, are also of the species. It is astonishing that on the water-colour Turner painted in 1802 after the woman of the double portrait in the Louvre (No. 1590), then known as Titian's mistress, the copyist should have grafted the Punch-like quality. It so happens that we have knowledge of Turner's long and compassionate devotion to but one person, his barber father who, for years a widower, acted as his son's factotum. (It is conceivable that there is an affinity, as Thornbury suggested, between some of Turner's figure-painting and barber's dummy heads that had probably once crowded his father's shop window in Maiden Lane.) F. E. Trimmer gave Thornbury this description of an unfinished portrait by Turner of his mother: 'There is a strong likeness to Turner about the nose and eyes. Her eyes are blue, lighter than his, her nose aquiline, and she has a slight fall in the nether lip. Her hair is well frizzed—for which she might have been in-debted to her husband's professional skill—and is sur-mounted by a cap with large flappers. She stands erect, and looks masculine, not to say fierce; report proclaims her to have been a person of ungovernable temper, and to have led her husband a sad life.' At the end of 1800, when Turner was twenty-five, his mother was taken to Bethlehem Hospital and discharged uncured the following year. She died in a private asylum in 1804. Other than the parentage, that is all we know of her.

Ruskin mentions Turner's favourite kind of declivity,

founded, Ruskin thinks, on his early Yorkshire studies, where he draws the precipitous part of hill or mountain in the lower section and a gradual slope on the top, a (phallic) formation that reverses the one typical in Rhine and Alps. When in 1792, at the age of seventeen, Turner recorded Magdalen bridge and tower at Oxford (T.B. 11), he worked from the bank below as he was so often to do in renderings of ruins, churches and castles. A strong towering above, a cascading below, were needed to give power to a delicate, almost pointilliste, drawing. The viewpoint was common enough, almost a convention, but we attribute to Turner an intoxication in its use since the imaginative range grew so wide in the treatment of wave, of masted ship and terraced, celestial palaces from whose thrust the sky but slowly withdraws its vapours. His first (1817) among several voyages to the Rhine with the crowd of precipitous castles, when he made drawings, and from them later, watercolours, will have particularly intensified a grasp of towering masses, natural and architectural, to which he had been long attracted; to which he could pin the utmost circumstance. Two years later Italian hill-towns impressed on him their broader affirmation: at that time he studied a variation he would always remember of the theme, the cascades, ravines, antique remains and ruins, propped among the prophetic trees of Tivoli. Before the end it ousted a stepped, orderly, Poussinesque type of composition such as we see in the superb, finished watercolour, *The Medway* (T.B. 208).

Turner's use of the old-fashioned viewpoint from above is more powerful still and more prevalent, the means of survey, of the bather's deliberate contemplation from the diving-board. We are given opportunity to linger there, and through our own volition we are thereupon immersed and enveloped by the scene. This appears, so often, a jump into our own past, heroically presented. The suspicion is surely strengthened if we consider subjects of his most ambitious work, fire and water, the disasters of fire and water or the wastes of ocean populated with giant fish and with the gestureless bodies from *The Slave Ship*, or by the near-swamped sailors of many a canvas such as the *Calais* and the *Trafalgar* or *The Shipwreck*, 1805. Not a few of Turner's predominant interests coalesced in Venice, boats, buildings, suffused by light and by the literary associations of Byron or Rogers, but a sea populated naturally, as it were, without shipwreck, a sea for the first time filled by people in a context without fury, since in Venice alone countless undistressed individuals are lying on the water, perhaps for *The Return from the Ball*. In his latter paintings of the city, Turner relaxed the piling-up trend of his phantasy: rush and fever subside into sad dreams of restless ease.

It is another miracle performed by that city. I must recall that the relationship to a part-object has the character of a complete identification, of a whirlpool envelopment into which we are drawn. Of such kind is Turner's more usual conception of doom and disaster, of the *Fallacies of Hope* (his poem, or pretended poem, from which he quoted in catalogues), the conception, in one aspect, of the infant who believes in the omnipotent and scalding propensity that belongs to his stream of yellow urine as it envelops the object so closely attached to himself, an object split off in his mind from the good breast with which he is also one. Whereas the two trends are integrated in Turner's art, he must emphasize with less vigour the long-studied separateness of self-sufficient and whole objects, other than as the pictures themselves, with a viewpoint, maybe, from above, now removed from the artist. The overall emphasis upon the canvas is predominantly the one of envelopment. We are likely to think first of late Turners in this connection. Though the approach be traditional the same quality is rarely absent from any but the earliest drawing and watercolour sketches. In a sketch-book of 1800-2 (T.B. 69) there are pastels on coarse blue paper one of which, a castle on a hill, presents but a pyramidal slab of slightly diaphanous colour, nearly of one tone. Though early oil set-pieces are particularly dark—eventually they lighten, first into greyness—and full of detail, they are not without a characteristic fluidity; hence, in all probability, Farington's description of 1796, 'mannered harmony'. After considerable and continuous success as a very young man, Turner's first great triumph was in 1801 with the Bridgewater sea-piece; already in 1802 (elected R.A.) he is accused of lack of finish; later, it will be of offering his public mere blotches. These, as a matter of fact, he kept to himself. In some cases, attributable mostly to the years 1820-30, of what Finberg in his Turner Bequest catalogue calls 'Colour Beginnings' watercolours (especially T.B. 263. There are also uncatalogued oil sketches), one is aware of experimentation with paint, yet of discoveries sufficient to themselves, though they can often be read without difficulty as first sketches in colour of landscapes and seascapes or as records of natural effects for which his memory was phenomenal. But it is impossible at this point, the crux of the Turner enigma, to remove his technical and aesthetic probing, probings into landscape design, from pressures anterior to them. All obsession has a vivid aspect of self-sufficiency. Anyone who looks through items, other than the earliest, of the vast Turner Bequest, will be amazed at the number of these 'beginnings' and pencil sketches, often monotonous in simplicity and sameness in regard to a raining downward of a top area upon a receptive area below: so many sheets in later times have no other feature, while others have a reverse surge from the lower section made up of vibrant stripes parallel to the picture plane, or of piercing forms as from an uneven sea. It appears that with the latter years, Turner brushed in large oil paintings for exhibition upon such preparations, sometimes their entirety as representations during the varnishing days. One element assaults the other in the simple,

zoned beginnings. Concentrating upon sky with land or sea, the
artist was under compulsion to record faithfully and repeat-
edly a stark intercourse, then to reconcile, then to interpose,
perhaps with a rainbow. Among the 'studies for vignettes'
of the 1830s (T.B. 280) there is a watercolour sheet of rose
with touches of ochre, saturated at the bottom, thin above.
Underneath this apparently abstract design of melting colour,
Turner has written—so runs the guess—'Sauve qui peut'.
It is to be expected that such delicate interplay of two
colours enfolded already for him the terrors of a flood,
equal to the chromatic balm in virtue of which the inevitable
alternation of the terror could be allowed to appear. With
comparable obsessiveness in his middle and final years,
Turner would draw rapidly a tower ensconced on a hill-top,
over and over again from every angle, perhaps six line-
drawings on one small page, doubtless with an eye to the best
design for a painting, but also to make far more than certain
from every long approach how the one element fitted into the
other: he often drew next day another tower and hill-top
with this fervour. An approximation, a drawing together, the
forging of an identity, so to say, out of evident differences as
is revealed by a fine use of colour, was a constant aim. In his
catalogue Finberg wrote of sketch-book 281 in the Turner
Bequest: 'A number of these pages have been prepared with
smudges of red and black watercolour, the colour then being
dabbed and rubbed, with the object apparently of producing
suggestions of figures, groups etc.' Maybe, but no figure or
group suggestions are to be seen, only the reconciliation of
the dense with the less dense. They resemble another common
type of beginning that is diaphanous and equal throughout.
For, naturally, rather than a prime imposition of contrast,
some coloured beginnings pre-eminently possess, like lay-ins,
the opposite or complementary value, that of the carver's
elicitation upon the stone's surface of a prevalent form
attributed to the block. Turner often used a rough blue or

grey paper on which his panoramic pencil drawings (even more than watercolouring) suggest messages that have appeared from within a wall upon its surface. An eloquent surface in this sense was integral to his art and became increasingly an influence upon its content. Divorced from that bent, his flamboyant confrontations would have lacked their union, the ease of interchange and coalescence, the issue of light, so often sunset, that floods.

In a region of the mind, as I have indicated, properties of fire and water (scalding) are not at variance but united, the hose of the fireman with the fire he inflames and, indeed, initiates. 'All his life,' wrote Kenneth Clark of Turner in passages to which I am much indebted, 'he had been obsessed by the conjunction of fire and water.' And: 'He loved the brilliance of steam, the dark diagonal of smoke blowing out of a tall chimney and the suggestion of hidden furnaces made visible at the mouth of a funnel.' Earlier, in *Landscape into Art*, Clark had a heading: 'Fire in the Flood', a quotation from *Beowulf*. 'Throughout the landscape of fantasy,' he wrote, 'it remains the painter's most powerful weapon, culminating in its glorious but extravagant use by Turner.' I think he enlarged upon fire in the flood far beyond this context of a Nature that was feared on every side in a dark and insecure age; it was a fear that must always have existed everywhere for irrational reasons alone, since there are bound to be phantasies of revengeful attacks issuing in kind from a scalded mother. Turner, it seems to me, largely denied this fear, pursued the attack but accepted the doom: he was possibly eager to discover those phantasies 'acted out' by a happening that he could represent as realism. In January 1792, when he was sixteen, he soon visited the burnt-out Pantheon in Oxford Street. A feature of his watercolour of the site next morning are icicles clinging to the façade, frozen water from the hoses. (In late life he attended to the processes of whaling—one instance is the boiling of blubber while

the boats are entangled by a flaw ice—and, of course, to giant
sea-monsters). It is the first occasion of which we know that
Turner's pencil, to use an expression of the time, was employed upon smouldering disaster. He was on the scene when
the Houses of Parliament were burning in 1834: he made
watercolour sketches and then two oil paintings: the sketches
are among his great masterpieces. Flames enwrap the high-
ways of the sky and of the Thames. Vessels coaling by torch-
light, *Keelmen heaving in Coals by Night*, is another lurid
canvas of this period. When he returned to Venice, probably
in 1835, he painted several sketches of rockets fired from
ships during a fiesta. A criticism of his *Juliet and Nurse*,
executed on his return, in which fireworks figure, was to the
effect that he made the night sky far too light. Another writer
said that *Juliet and Nurse* was nothing more than a further
conflagration of the Houses of Parliament. Turner exhibited
in 1832 *Nebuchadnezzar at the Mouth of the fiery Furnace*.
'Fire' or 'Heat' and 'Blood' were words commonly used in
contemporary writing on him. It is surely unnecessary to
remark, in respect to fire and water, the many watery sunrises
and bloody sunsets or *Rain, Steam and Speed* and *Fire at Sea*.
Turner himself wrote 'Fire and Blood' in the sky of a drawing
that may be dated 1806-8 (T.B. 101). The onrush of ivy, and
other leafage in his best architectural drawings are profoundly related with effects of rock and water such as the
wonderful watercolour of 1795, *Melincourt Fall*, where the
unbroken slab or wedge of water licks the fractured rock
like a flame. Soon after reaching Rome for the first time in
October 1819, Turner hurried to Naples where Vesuvius
had become active some days before.

Allied with the one of fire there is often conveyed by his
work a sense of explosion, in the famous *Snowstorm*
(exhibited 1842), for instance, or even in the earlier snowstorm of *Hannibal crossing the Alps* of 1812. One sees from
afar an atmosphere of paint and detonation, then one searches

for the benighted human beings who, when found, remark the processes of meteorological might rather than of individuals who endure them. On the other hand, Olympic vistas, calm temples, survive in our general impression of Turner's art: in view of a ceaseless lyrical bias it is a humane art. We learn from him that calamity is asymmetrical.

Ruskin deplored Turner's lack of interest in the detail of Gothic architecture (despite the numerous, astounding studies of, say, Rouen cathedral). A brooding attachment to the classical orders is strangely suggested by bawdy lines he wrote eroticizing the Ionic. (It is not altogether surprising to discover there a punning use of words that could reflect the infantile oral phantasy of the *vagina dentata*.)

In connection with my mention of scalding attacks I think it relevant to remark Turner's liberal use of yellows. *Dido building Carthage* was originally thought too yellow. Turner himself writes to a friend in 1826: 'I must not say yellow, for I have taken it *all* to my keeping this year, so they say.' And later that year: 'Callcott is going to be married to an acquaintance of mine when in Italy, a very agreeable Blue Stocking, so I must wear the yellow stockings.' Rippingille reported from Rome a *mot* about a retailer of English mustard who was coupled with Turner: 'The one sold mustard, the other painted it.' 'A devil of a lot of chrome' is how Scarlett Davis described to Ince the *Burning of the House of Lords and Commons*. (Van Gogh, a more aggressive handler of everything fiery, and his passion for yellow, are better known today.)

I find it fair to say that the compulsively unitary, forcing side of Turner's art strengthened, indeed largely inspired, a further linking by his late paintings of elements already long harmonized through the delicacy of his touch, through his heightened sense of texture and colour relationship, a building, for instance, and its foliage, the structure and its attenuations, what is rough with what is smooth, the perpendicular

68

with the transverse by means of the ellipse. I have emphasized primitive and aggressive compulsions in Turner's art, but I have wanted to suggest that in admitting them, in giving due place to ferocity and the consequent despair, his very powerful lyrical vein was not impaired: throughout his oeuvre it was enriched: in many, very many, supremely lyrical works, a linking, a co-ordination, an integration, of different degrees of compulsion and different tendencies of the mind were achieved. In the great last period, not only is the world washed clean by light, but humidity is sucked from water, the core of fire from flame, leaving an iridescence through which we witness an object's ceremonious identity: whereupon space and light envelop them and us, cement the world under the aegis of a boat at dawn between Cumaean headlands, or a yacht that gains the coast.

Together with Turner's whirlpool of fire and water we experience beneficence in space. There abound calm scenes that would be sombre or forlorn without the gold, without the agitated pulse and delicacy in so light a key.

Beneficence is very widely scattered; encompasses from afar.

Turner's accomplishment, so large, so various, easily falsifies an investigation whose author singles out this or that upon which to base appreciation, as I have done after studying the several thousand sketches in water- or body-colour, the countless pencil drawings (British Museum) of the Turner Bequest and the near 300 oils (Tate Gallery).

There is abundant evidence, for instance, to show that Turner could both record and improvise figures or groups in any attitude and in a variety of styles. His sketch-books reveal that he was attracted by crowded scenes and new forms of animation. On first visiting Edinburgh he, most unusually, almost filled a sketch-book with figures, largely the girls with giant shawls and bare feet. It was much the same during his first visit to Holland in 1817 and to Switzerland in 1802: on the first page of T.B. 78 there is a watercolour of two nude girls on a bed. The watercolour he exhibited in 1799, *Inside the Chapter House of Salisbury Cathedral*, contains figures on the floor about a pillar, youths and a girl, realized with very apt draughtmanship. If brilliance in this genre be not uncommon, if in his watercolours an adequacy for figures is the rule, it seems the more reasonable to remark as most significant the wooden and childlike element in the presentation of some of Turner's crowds especially, though this quality is not shared by a later group of oil figure compositions, such as *Rembrandt's Daughter reading a Love-Letter* (exhib. 1827) or *Watteau Study* and *Lord Percy under Attainder* (1831) nor by an earlier history or myth painting such as *The Garden of Hesperides* (1806) or the *Macon* of 1803. Nor is it shared by his rapid figure sketches, though they fall short of a corresponding calligraphy for landscape and architectural jotting, of sublime notations too for crowded shipping with masts (e.g. T.B. 206 & 226). On the other hand, feminine fashion that emphasized an answering slope of bare shoulders and the pin of the head, fired Turner's droll, unflinching portraits. Even though earlier landscape and genre masters had been content to offer no more than an abrupt consort of lay figures, it is surely interesting that one of the most facile, as well as the most imaginative, of artists whose forte was the rendering of fluidity (apparent even in these portraits), should, in the course of development, have sometimes populated the seas and declivities of vast canvases with variegated dolls. I therefore offered in the earlier part of this essay psychological interpretations that so far from increasing the contrast, sought to unify a fluidity in handling Nature with part-object, doll- or Punch-like conceptions, a viewpoint that might allow us to discern the aspect of Turner's genius wherein an evident compulsive element, close, at times, to the childlike, was not ousted by his manifold abilities

nor by an extremely professional *savoir faire*. He found a
way to employ the whole of himself, the immature as well as
the mature and to fit them together. First he was the complete
servant of the art taught to him, the art and culture of his
contemporaries and predecessors. (As late as 1821 Turner
was bidding at a sale for sketch-books, with notes on Old
Masters, by Reynolds.) Meanwhile and thereafter, in the
interests of wider co-ordination, he continued to amplify
the resources of his own nature, as of Nature outside, for an
aesthetic purpose.

I contrasted very cursorily what appears in Turner's case
an ideal evolution, with the dilemma of the art student today.
It was said of Turner's later exhibited oils that it had no
bearing on an impression of soap-suds or poached eggs that
the title of a painting read 'Whalers' or 'Venice': the scene
was unrecognizable, the picture ever the same. But 'pictures
of nothing, and very like' was Hazlitt's famous criticism
as early as 1816. It could be said to have a witty pertinence
to a few 'extreme' canvases that Turner would be painting
some twenty or thirty years later, though not in one instance
of work carried through, are we in doubt as to the type of
subject. Hazlitt's stricture on the exhibited paintings of 1816
and before can be comprehended only in the historical
setting.

Even in a very late 'all-over' painting—others, the watercolour exemplars, had dared it only on a small scale—that
at first sight seems abstract, since it is featureless in regard to
vertical shapes, in the last sea-scapes, for instance, at the
Tate, we acknowledge almost immediately that here is a
record, an intense record, of an outward as well as an inward
scene: we are aware that in virtue of familiarity, detail has
been undone by a virtuoso performer who, conscious of
power and information, has no fear of too great a freedom
that might result in an overriding of the object and cause
the artist to construct shapes, to use colours, dictated solely

F   71

by his design. Turner's reverence for the objects he studied was intact. He employed freedom to realize movement, depth and interaction, without major recourse to the arbitrary. He has seemed to relax where, in reality, he has broken down or eschewed trite constructions in himself as in the object after long apprenticeship and ceaseless observation.

According to Hazlitt, Turner was more concerned with the mediums—the light—in which things appear than with the localized aspect of those things themselves. He wrote: 'The artist (Turner) delights to go back to the first chaos of the world.' These words suggest not only subsequent canvases such as *Morning after the Deluge* (exhib. 1843), but also the thunderous calm implicit in an unravelled golden mist that characterizes many earlier classical subjects and *Crossing the Brook* (exhib. 1815). I would prefer to say that inspired with traditional poetic feeling, he was rehearsing the chief relationships of the psyche to its objects, particularly an enveloping relationship associated with the breast. In the late or extreme 'all-over' oil paintings, liquid and light-toned, we sense more easily what might be called a breathing or palpitation of the sky, water and land: touches of contrasting colour, scattered masses, seem to furnish a source for the nurture of this ambience, a treatment evident in some drawings and sketches of all periods except the first, from which—and from the best of the earlier English watercolour school—these oils eventually derive. A light, pulsating, ambience where buildings are sometimes treated almost as clouds (*The Piazzetta; Venice*) makes possible the accomplishment within the key of a startling foreground relief, or of masses lying back, in the Venetian Ball paintings, for instance, or in *Norham Castle: Sunrise*, the most beautiful.

Once more, the late Turner exists in some aspects of the earlier work. For instance, *Kilgarran Castle*, exhibited at the Royal Academy in 1799, projects, under the influence of Wilson, flanking hill-clumps and a towering yet misty or enveloping distance. Clumps and iridescent clefts become an unavoidable jargon; they provide the principle of most of the early sea- and subsequent estuary-pieces; they are allegories for feminine form and function, but often a base as well for the element of counterpoint, for a union of directions and oppositions, for the fusion of *The Sun rising through Vapour*, if I may instance the title, in addition to the famous painting itself. By means of low sun or moon in low sky, Turner has furnished in his studies an expanded world, soft, vaporous yet certain, not once but a hundred times.

I must enlarge upon clefts and clumps before referring to the counterpoint. If these be allegories of feminine form and function as a whole, yet the nuzzling, the enveloping, the part-object symbolism, is their stronger facet, so often dramatized in representations of vast space, by Turner's own small figure also, in top-hat and tail-coat (*vide* the Parrott portrait) with nose almost pressing it as he works a considerable canvas at the Academy or British Institution, without stepping back. Though it is written by an artist who was usually hostile and malevolent about Turner, some of the account, confirmed in the main elsewhere, is worth remark of Turner and his *Burning of the House of Lords and Commons* on a varnishing day, 1835, at the British Institution. 'He was there at work', wrote E. V. Rippingille in a reminiscence of Callcott (*Art Journal* 1860), 'Before I came, having set to work at the earliest hour allowed. Indeed it was quite necessary to make the best of his time, as the picture when sent in was a mere dab of several colours, and 'without form and void' (Hazlitt), like chaos before the creation. . . ' Etty was working at his side (on his picture *The Lute Player*) . . . 'Little Etty stepped back every now and then to look at the effect of his picture, lolling his head on one side and half-closing his eyes, and sometimes speaking to someone near him, after the approved manner of painters: but not so Turner; for the three hours I was there—and I understood it had been the same since he

F*   73

began in the morning—he never ceased to work, or even once looked or turned from the wall on which his picture hung. All lookers-on were amused by the figure Turner exhibited in himself, and the process he was pursuing with his picture . . . Leaning forward and sideways over to the the right, the left-hand metal button of his blue coat rose six inches higher than the right, and his head buried in his shoulders and held down, presented an aspect curious to all beholders . . . Presently the work was finished: Turner gathered up his tools together, put them into and shut up the box, and then, with his face still turned to the wall, and at the same distance from it, went sideling off, without speaking a word to anybody.'

We can take it that in the act of painting, even his vast distances were pressed up against the visionary eye like the breast upon the mouth: at the same time it was he who fed the infant picture. In these embracing conceptions, no wonder that figures glue themselves on banks and bases, variegated figures, salmon-like, dully flashing films of colour, perhaps floating beneath a cloud-like architecture, perhaps pressed to the ground like the catch in baskets upon a quay, glistening at dawn. Ruskin remarked on the accumulations of bric-à-brac in Turnerian foregrounds—I would include bodies and jetsam in seas, or on an earth so flattened in some late canvases as to suggest a pavement of rippled water—and referred them to the grand confusion of Covent Garden where Turner lived as a child. An equation persists, as is well known, between nipple and phallus. The above description of Turner at work in 1835 at the British Institution may recall the couplet twice used in his incomprehensible verses entitled *The Origin of Vermilion or the Loves of Painting and Music*:

> *As snails trail o'er the morning dew*
> *He thus the line of beauty drew.*

He sought daring expedients for his sense of fitness: in

74

the case of persons especially, I repeat, they were based on part-object models. The companions, the siblings, he projected, are often like shoals; as mere members, as mouths perhaps, they may flit about the declivities and rises of an encompassing breast, much of it out of reach as palace, torrent, ocean, mountain or murderous sky.

No wonder Turner criticized Poussin's *Deluge* in the Louvre for lack of 'current and ebullition' in the water, though he was much influenced by Poussin at that time (1802). Ruskin wrote as follows for the first volume of *Modern Painters* about *The Slave Ship*: 'The whole surface of the sea is divided into two ridges of enormous swell, not high, not local, but a low broad heaving of the whole ocean, like the lifting of its bosom by deep-drawn breath after the torture of the storm.'

These are mounds, clumps, of terror and benignity; within one of the shapes, a pyramid of pearly monsters has been confounded with the black, disappearing bodies. The pyramid of *Fire at Sea*, huge, massive, is thrown upwards against a mound of cloud. Swart, irregular pyramids characterize the famous *Snowstorm* whose ship is like a broken caterpillar, whereas the engulfed mariners of *Fire at Sea* are near to having become, as if protectively, globular, saffron-coloured fish. A subject for Turner's attention, particularly in the neighbourhood of Plymouth during 1811, as numerous drawings and two canvases at Petworth testify, lay with the tall curving ribs of naval hulks, ruined globes of timber, derelict hills that rode upon the Tamar. The *Téméraire* would later achieve amid sunset fires superb apotheosis for hulks, unruined, full of distance from the funnelled infant steamboat by which it is tugged, to which it is closely attached.

It would be tedious to enumerate the recurrence of a fluidity that possesses clumps, mounds, pyramids and clefts, though I am fascinated by this theme, especially in paintings that Turner showed at his last Academy of 1850, *Visit to the Tomb* and *Departure of the Trojan Fleet*, among his ultimate Punic paintings. I must remark the extraordinary volume of such unmoored shapes, since there was earlier mention of poorness of relief in another context. Had he been primarily a figure painter—in this matter it is no contradiction to imagine so—Turner would have attained poignant compositions in terms of that theme: the so-called *Costume Piece* at the Tate suggests it.

To summarize Turner's clump or mound conception would be, I think, to isolate a parting of the ways, a rustling or seething withdrawal as in the biblical passage of the Red Sea: to many mythological scenes an opalescent, warm passage is common through the centre, and on one side, maybe, the silent arm of a tall pine.

It remains to speak of the tension, the counterpoint, the bringing together of storm with sun, disaster with beauty, melancholy with protected ease in many, many, parkland expanses, and, in general, the good with the bad. Formal contrivances that suggest their union are not of course themselves symbolic in the immediate conscious sense of the rainbow, for instance, of the *Wreck Buoy*. More significant, however, even here (as deep-laid symbol), the high, lit, sail-tops, ghostly against a sky that falls in curtains of rain, cleave to the rainbow's half-circle triangularly, in contrast with foreground water, wastes rich in light flanked by darker mounds of sea, that topple over towards the spectator yet seem at the back to climb up to the boats and to the falling sky. The meeting of these movements occurs near the centre of the canvas from where one has the sense of extracting the heart of so vertiginous, so desert, yet so various a scene, in terms of the red-rose jib on the nearer sailing boat: at either side verticals incline outwards and thereby stress that centre. Awareness of a centre in great space will favour a *rencontre* of contrary factors in whatever sense. Turner was no stranger to the manipulation and perhaps even to the confusion of contrary factors. I cannot help remarking, as shown to me by B. A. R. Carter, that two demonstration sheets, illustrating a triangle fitted into a circle, that he used for his Perspective lectures, are each headed 'Circle (or circles) within a Triangle'.

A motif more constant in the work of Turner even than the one of clumps with their clefts, is the rhythmic use of a rebuttal, very commonly of waves blown back as they break on a lea shore, apparent already in early sea-pieces and in mountain brooks whose drums of shallow water rolling over boulders provide the effect of a reversing power, a break. He often represents the force of natural agency by demonstrating that it is engaged, sometimes thwarted by another. *The Falls of Terni* drop as one body, then are broken, buffetted. A stoic pathos, inherent in the beauty, sustains those great last light canvases wherein hardly a boat interrupts the grappling of sea with sky, wherein naked oppositions and their reconciliation supply overall bareness to the opulence of the effect. Yet even in narrow paintings of flat scenes, *Chichester Canal* or *Petworth Park with Tillington Church in the distance* (sketches at the Tate for the Petworth landscapes), at the meeting of ground and sky there is the effect of a scooped-out pomegranate or apricot common to the pictures of Petworth interiors, a benign application of the whirlwind principle, at the picture's centre, at the centre of interest. (The theme is at least as old as exquisite studies for *The Sun rising through Vapour*). Maybe a low sun is there to help us seize upon the otherwise faintly indicated fruit, both soft and fierce, romantic in promise as in muted danger and elusive distance. Amid the embraces of hugeness, we have seen that figuration, men more than cattle, are sometimes a startling variant, like fossil traces that vivify a rock. The infant's experiences have been similarly engraved by him upon the sudden breast.

Clasping natural immensity, Turner lent a hard-won grandeur to the distance, so irregularly spanned by each of us, between self-destruction and forgetful, infantile love.

As he elaborates an insight conditioned by his time, the artist, I have supposed in the first essay, may project images that need not correspond altogether with his most native bent. Naturally, the correspondence will have been very close in the case of superb individualists. All the same, it is impossible even to guess how potently Turner's uniqueness could have survived abstraction from the historical context, and it is impossible to know how deeply, how widely, the primitive obsessions that were exploited by his art, qualified the structure of his ego. In making an end, therefore, not only to this brief examination of his peculiar genius but also to wider issues in this book, a word or two are required for the other side of the balance.

A broad issue has been the artist's ambivalence, the bringing together he imposes on it. Turner pre-eminently dramatized that *rencontre* when he applied it to a state where it does not truly belong, to the earlier emotions of over-powering alternations before ambivalence has been admitted, embracing the then current notions of 'the sublime', of what is rapturous, transporting yet often vast and terrible, in a word, enveloping. Through chromatic wealth, through the brilliant identity between great differences that colour can create, an equation habitually survives in Turner's major work between dissolution, disruption and suave continuity, between richness and the bareness of distance: neither term suffers from their union; neither is overlaid, disguised. While light that dominates so many of his landscapes is rich and bounteous, it obliterates also, flooding building, water and mountain to the length, sometimes, of their near-extinction. Accepting his sublimity, entertaining thus a merging experience, the spectator shrinks as a complete or separate entity but regains himself as he absorbs the stable self-inclusiveness of the art object.

Now, an open landscape or sea-scape will sometimes induce the first part of this affect more fully than the second: the artist's treatment of such a landscape, not only Turner's, often disposes shapes that I have called breast-like clumps. What he developed from this arrangement in a light key is unique, but Turner was much under the influence of Wilson when, as a young man, he painted *Coniston Falls*, exhibited in 1798; the picture shows a grouping of masses typical of Turner's late canvases.

The Romantic Movement as a whole welcomed an equation between an envelopment through a state of nurture and through the ungovernable moods, the overpowering forces of Nature. The long reach of the inner life, particularly in an infantile form, when projected on to Nature, directed Wordsworthian pantheism. The Romantic Movement had been preceded by the speculation of a century upon the character of 'the sublime', in the case of art upon some feasible irregularity or excess intruding within the well-controlled relationships of an acknowledged tempo. In the later part especially of this period there was also an attention to Nature where she herself suggests the interlocking attributes of a painting; to the picturesque. This was an aspect, discussed by Richard Payne Knight at least (in whose company J. R. Cozens probably made his first journey to Italy in 1776) as independent to some extent of association, as 'merely visible beauty abstracted from all mental sympathies or intellectual fitness' (*An Analytical Inquiry into the Principles of Taste*, 2nd edition, 1805). Though Knight had restricted his pure qualities of vision to those of light and colour, this early version of 'significant form' calls to mind particularly Francis Towne's and Cotman's best work where they have concentrated without ado upon the bones of structure. The forms even of the Campagna landscape predominate, in the hands of the two Cozens, not only over details of antique remains but over elegiac or pastoral associations.

Their drawings and watercolours communicate emotion, albeit poetic emotion, more generally. 'Cozens (J.R.) is all poetry', said Constable who described him as 'the greatest artist who ever touched landscape'. Many monochrome or wash drawings at the turn of the century, such as the blue wash drawings of evening common to Girtin, Turner and Cotman, are closely related to his work (Oppé). For three years, probably from 1794-7, Girtin and Turner were employed by Dr. Monro to trace and then colour after J.R. Cozens (among others). Mountains are hardly more substantial than the clouds in many Cozens' wash drawings, such is their poetic accent upon breadth and homogeneity. Alexander Cozens, the father, had insisted 'that the true character of a subject lay in its boldest and broadest aspect' (Oppé). As in the work of the non-literary Girtin later, precept for his compositions was based less upon old pictures or literary association than upon the categories of landscape itself. Alexander Cozens devised a system for unravelling compositions from blots made boldly with a brush while an idea of landscape was present in the mind (*A New Method of Assisting the Invention in Drawing original Compositions of Landscape*, 1786. More than one story about Turner shows that his procedure had not been forgotten. cf. Hamerton). Brought up in Russia he may have seen monochrome, free flowing, examples of Far Eastern brushwork. We know that he was given a sheet of calligraphic Persian drawings in St. Petersburg: it passed into his patron's, Beckford's, possession. It is most likely that Turner examined major work by both Cozens when he was at Fonthill in 1799. He will have noted the slowly insistent (rather than rapid or sketch-like) breadth of treatment in a finished, long-worked watercolour, this the only contribution ever made by English painters to a broad or grand manner all their own, a manner enlarged at times by Girtin with the invention of a more direct attack, bound up with better papers and new colours, by Cotman and, throughout, vastly by Turner who, at the same time, neither spurned a combination with an imaginative, literary approach nor lost his zest pursuing a far wider public by means of continuous engraving.

These very few references are sufficient to remind the reader concerning the danger, a necessity of so short a statement, of treating an artist for one moment in isolation.

But of course the greatness of Turner lies not only in his opportunity and in his temperament adapted to it. 'Turner was gifted,' wrote Laurence Binyon, 'with a hand and eye of incomparable delicacy; he had an amazing visual memory, an inexhaustible appetite for observation of the subtlest kind. He was immensely ambitious, and his ambition was equalled by his patience and docility. By nature close and secretive, he was bent on learning and never ceased to learn, ready to take hints from any of the masters, while accumulating within his mind store upon store of first-hand knowledge through his eyesight.' Yet it must be added that at least some of these propensities and of this application might have been withheld from art under different cultural conditions. In the event, no other English artist has been so deeply, so intelligently, informed of Nature as well as of the Masters. 'The sense of England,' wrote Binyon, 'which pervades the drawings of his youth and early manhood has expanded into a sense of Europe: but in the end this also merges into something wider and profounder, a sense of the whole related universe.' I would add that this 'universe' serves to reflect strongly what I have called the inner life, particularly the inner life at a very early and comparatively simple level.

But amid every febrile deployment Turner kept his head. 'One marvels,' says Binyon, 'at . . . the evocation of complex forms, however submerged in aerial hues, the fullness of the distances. It is the same with the Alpine scenes, where the mountains retain their sculptured form yet seem built of light and air.'

Maybe Binyon had particularly in mind chosen water-colour sketches—there was still a gap between sketches and work commissioned from them—allotted to the early 1840s, some, for instance, of Lucerne lake and its surroundings (where Cozens too had excelled). I consider these latter-day lake watercolours—not of Lucerne only—to be Turner's crowning achievement, and therefore the best things by an English painter. With their height, reduplication and reflection below, the Alps were translated into infectious forms of stupendous chromatic beauty. What Cézanne would later achieve before the brow of Mont Saint-Victoire, Turner lavished finally in a few small-scale works upon endless, enfolding prospects.

Turner integrated eccentricity with the demands of adulthood: in the situation of successful creativeness, we have seen, compulsion and obsession need not debar breadth: nor did they in Turner's life. Miserly and extortionate with small money, acquisitive of culture, he commanded many generous feelings and wide interests. He was always very loyal, particularly to his parents, to their want or poverty. Gruff, kind to children and to many others; morose, cheerless in a preferred shabbiness, dry of humour, he often enjoyed company away from home. He was astute not only in his own business but over the Academy's business to which he gave much time in association with others. Often a recluse, we know he suffered deeply on the death of his friends. Unregenerated by ridicule, in seeking what he felt he remained without veneer. His painting of set-pieces enshrines under fustian an incorrigible body of primitive vision, transforming an eighteenth-century argot for grandiloquent nostalgia into epics of naked need, subordinating rhetoric to an unbroken immediacy attributed to Nature, unbroken, however refurbished; and therefore unbroken rather than refurbished. Hard, not to say cruel, in the requirement from engravers, he caused them to become the best in Europe. A very rich self-made man, he spent £3,000 buying back plates, lest they fall into inferior hands; yet unwanted masterpieces, and those he had himself bought back at huge prices—he meant all to go to the nation—rotted in a damp gallery, often sure to lose colour due to impulsive techniques. As well as supreme goodness, he will have attributed to his accumulated canvases a corruptible aspect that swelled his sense of loss and decay.

In his later years there is an episode that seems the happiest. Not long after the death of his father in the autumn of 1829, he appears to have spent much time with Lord Egremont at Petworth, occupying a studio. Rothenstein and Butlin have written of the 'liberation' of his colour in the luminous interiors he is thought to have executed there, remarking that it is strange that this even bolder attack should be realized first in figure scenes such as the studies of music-making, rather than through his landscapes.

I hazard the guess that under the aegis of the unpretentious, far-seeing Egremont and his vast collection, the early Turner household, together with an accumulation of artefacts dating from the crowded Covent Garden days, were momentarily reconstituted in a monumental and perfected version, in a version, as it were, of classic stone. Not only are the landscapes that Turner then painted for Petworth among his greatest and calmest, but in the subject-picture sketches, in the interiors, he was approaching nearer—also Rothenstein and Butlin remark it—than at any time we know of since his self-portrait as a youth, to a colourful appreciation through his art of entire human beings, at any rate of his companions rather than of strangers. There are signs in a few drawings of the late twenties of such a development; it is heralded by the *Jessica* he had painted during the second Roman visit; a development encouraged by Egremont inasmuch as he bought *Jessica*. The famous *Interior at*

Petworth whose scattering chromatic lights disperse, dispense with, bric-à-brac, animals, birds in the grandeur of a hall, may mark, as has been suggested by David Thomas for barely discernible iconographic reasons, Egremont's death in 1837, and so the completion of this happier phase.

Turner died in 1851 at the age of seventy-six, in a small cottage on the river bank at Chelsea, as far as his surgeon and, presumably, his neighbours were concerned, under the name of Booth, the one of his widowed housekeeper there.

Some References

BINYON, L. *English Water-Colours* (London, 1933).

BELL, C. F. *A List of the Works contributed to Public Exhibitions by J. M. W. Turner, R.A.* (London, 1901).

BELL, C. F. and GIRTIN, T. *The Drawings and Sketches of John Robert Cozens* (Walpole Society, 1935).

BURNET, J. and CUNNINGHAM, P. *Turner and his Works* (London, 1852).

BUTLIN, M. *The Watercolours of J. M. W. Turner* (London, 1962).

CLARE, C. *J. M. W. Turner* (London, 1951).

CLARK, K. *Landscape into Art* (London, 1949).

CLARK, K. *Looking at Pictures* (London, 1960).

CROFT MURRAY, E. 'Pencil Outlines of Shipping at Dover of the Monro School' (*B.M. Quarterly*, Vol. X).

FINBERG, A. J. *Complete Inventory of the Drawings of the Turner Bequest.* 2 Vols (London, 1910).

FINBERG, A. J. *Turner's Sketches and Drawings* (London, 1910).

FINBERG, A. J. *In Venice with Turner* (London, 1930).

FINBERG, A. J. *The Life of J. M. W. Turner, R.A.* (London, 1939 and 1961).

GIRTIN, T. and LOSHAK, D. *The Art of Thomas Girtin* (London, 1954).

HAMERTON, P. G. *The Life of J. M. W. Turner, R.A.* (London, 1895).

HUSSEY, C. *The Picturesque* (London, 1927).

LIVERMORE, A. N. 'Turner and Music' (*Music and Letters*, 1957).

LIVERMORE, A. N. 'Turner's Unknown Verse-book' (*Connoisseur Year Book*, 1957).

MONK, S. H. *The Sublime. A Study of Critical Theories in 18th Century England* (Michigan, 1935 and 1960).

OPPÉ, A. P. *Alexander and John Robert Cozens* (London, 1952).

ROTHENSTEIN, J. and BUTLIN, M. *Turner* (London, 1963).

RUSKIN, J. *Works* (Vols. 3-7, *Modern Painters*, Library Edition).

RUSKIN, J. *Notes by Mr. Ruskin on his Collection of Drawings by the late J. M. W. Turner, R.A.* (London, 1878).

THORNBURY, W. *Life of J. M. W. Turner, R.A.* (2 vols. London, 1862).

TURNER, J. M. W. *Verse Book MS.* (in collection of Charles M. W. Turner, Esq.)

Index